ART & ANATOMY:

DRAWINGS

ART & ANATOMY: DRAWINGS

Master Scholars Program in Humanistic Medicine, New York University School of Medicine

This publication was supported in part by a grant from the Louis and Rachel Rudin Foundation, Inc.

Published by University of California Medical Humanities Press

ISBN 979-0-9963242-5-0

Library of Congress Control Number: 2017958269

Front cover artwork: Hannah Bernstein, "Open Heart"

Printed in Canada

ART & ANATOMY:
DRAWINGS

Laura Ferguson & Katie Grogan, Editors

Master Scholars Program in Humanistic Medicine,

New York University School of Medicine

Foreword by Danielle Ofri, MD, PhD

University of California Medical Humanities Press

ART & ANATOMY is a seminar in the
Master Scholars Program in Humanistic Medicine
at the New York University School of Medicine.

The artists are medical students, physicians, health professionals,
researchers, and staff from across NYU Langone Health at all levels,
from beginning to accomplished.

They made the drawings in this book over an eight-year period from the
seminar's founding in 2009 to the present.

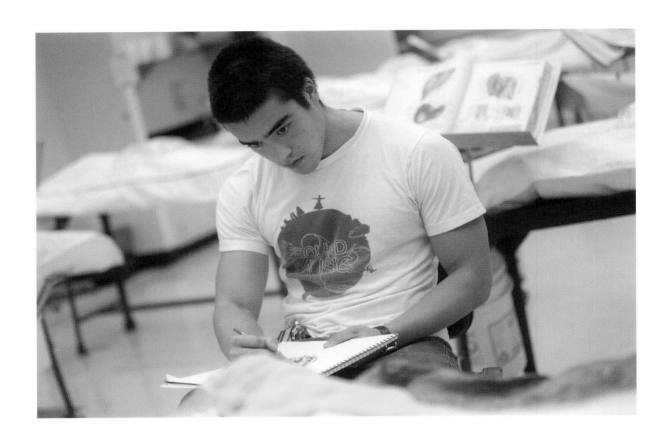

The Art of Medicine

Foreword by Danielle Ofri, MD, PhD

"Artistic" isn't the first descriptor that comes to mind when entering the anatomy lab. Stuffy, smelly, drippy, disgusting are more common adjectives. But every medical student is issued a guide upon entering this strange world. For me, my Virgil was Grant's *Atlas of Anatomy*. I affixed a plastic cover over it in a vain effort to keep it clean, but the pages inevitably became crinkled from formalin, stained from juices of preferably uninvestigated origin, and gristled from sweaty hands desperately trying to divine the enigmatic roadmap of the human body.

The technical instructions in the atlas were a godsend, but I was most taken with the drawings. In an era when photographic exactitude or computer rendering could have provided perfect similitude, the authors of this book and other comparable atlases chose to offer drawings. These grayscale drawings rendered the human body in exquisite intimate detail. Thinking back to this now, I realize that what entranced me about these drawings was that I could imagine a person actually drawing them. When the picture showed forceps deferentially moving aside a muscle to reveal the delicate underlying vasculature, I could envision one hand of the artist holding those forceps, while the other furiously sketched the treasure beneath.

Anatomy atlases created from CT or MRI images didn't elicit the same response in me. Those books were helpful, to be sure, but they felt impersonal, objective. I didn't have any sense of anyone "doing" those images, though I certainly knew there had to be actual humans running the machines and creating the books.

But the drawings of Grant's *Atlas* and Gray's *Anatomy* and the brilliantly colored Netter books all retained traces of the human hand, traces of the artist. I could picture the authors separating viscera with their (hopefully) gloved hands, all the while considering how best they could bring to life—as it were—the dead who lay before them.

Artists, of course, have always strived to bring their subjects to life on the canvas and the human figure remains the most challenging subject. But the desire to delve beneath the skin is a particular blend of scientific drive and esthetic rigor.

This combination was clearly on display when Renaissance physician Andreas Vesalius published his *De humani corporis fabrica* in 1543. Having honed his dissection skills on the corpses of executed criminals, he sought to transmit this knowledge visually in a seven-volume series that was an immediate best-seller.

Vesalius's primary contribution to anatomy was accuracy. For the preceding millennium, physicians relied on the flawed descriptions of Galen, who had based his knowledge on animal dissection and his own intuition. Vesalius instead worked from direct observation of human cadavers. But *De humani corporis fabrica* was equally famed for its artistic skill and sense of style. Simply transcribing what he saw was not enough for Vesalius. He directed the artists he worked with to set their human figures in the sylvan countryside. Villages, church steeples, rolling hills, rivers, and bridges appear in the background.

Even more dramatically, the figures were shown in action, often in agony. As layers of muscles are peeled off, the bodies droop from lack of support. Knees buckle and torsos keel. Heads loll—sometimes from dissected musculature, other times from a hangman's noose. Heads end up in the palm of the hand, though not before a clean transverse slicing of the cranium to reveal the inner ventricles.

Even the bare skeletons appear capable of conveying emotion. Vesalius's skeletons seem to express contemplation, anguish, despair. Inspiring his artists to the heights of creativity, Vesalius produced a masterpiece of anatomical artistry.

Sixty years before Vesalius burst onto the scene, however, another artist was hard at work with his own vivid and accurate anatomical drawings. In the late 1480s, Leonardo da Vinci obtained a human skull. Fascinated by this ornate natural sculpture, he began a series of anatomical drawings of the skull, apparently planning a magnum opus of the human body. But either he didn't have access to more human material or he simply got caught up in a myriad of commissions, because another fifteen years went by before he returned to human anatomy.

When he did return, though, he had access to full-body cadavers and thus set out to chart the entire human body. As a consummate scientist-artist, Leonardo was as concerned with discerning the way the body worked as with how the body should be rendered. While it's impossible to conjecture motivation, one might imagine how the exquisite beauty of the body's undercarriage propelled the scientific scrutiny.

Leonardo's resultant output was a tour de force of the human body. He indubitably produced the first anatomically accurate rendering. His cross-sectional "cuts" and multiple points-of-view presaged modern anatomical teachings. Additionally, he elucidated much of its physiology, most notably of the heart. He elucidated the four-chamber structure, the conical pumping of the heart and the intricate functioning of the aortic valve.

His drawings and explanations would have been sufficient to unseat the thousand-year reign of Galen's erroneous theories. Yet Leonardo chose not to publish his work. His revolutionary ideas and art sat untouched. Vesalius reached many of the same conclusions—at least anatomically—a half-century later. But because of Leonardo's earlier silence, Vesalius became the one who toppled Galen.

It's not clear exactly why Leonardo did not publish his seminal drawings. It may have been due to the political turmoil in Milan, or the abrupt death (from bubonic plague) of his sometime anatomy partner

Marcantonio della Torre, or simply that he got sidetracked into other intriguing ventures such as elucidating embryology, designing wells, or painting landscapes. Whatever the case, his more than 700 groundbreaking drawings, and countless notes remained essentially unknown to the greater world for some 500 years.

Some scholars speculate that Leonardo may have made a conscious decision to keep his drawings private. (His frequent habit of mirror-writing might have been an active method to keep his work to himself). One wonders if Leonardo might have been more actively focused on the process of learning and drawing rather than on the product of these endeavors.

We the public are grateful that at least some of his product finally saw the light of day, but there is much to be gained by concentrating on the process. The drawings in the book before you are a result of the attention to process.

The medical students who participated in Art & Anatomy were not training to become artists, but rather taking their first steps toward becoming physicians. Spending extra time with patients, even deceased ones, is crucial for developing the doctor-patient connection. Learning the ins and outs of patients—physically and emotionally—are all part of the process of becoming an astute physician. Developing creativity and sensitivity is necessary to transform a doctor who is smart into a doctor who is wise.

Medical training is typically a frenzied affair, with vast tracts of knowledge bulldozing their way into the minds of students at a tumultuous pace. One thing students rarely have the opportunity for is contemplation. Art & Anatomy is one of the few oases within medical school where time and space are carved out for this. The photos in this book portray the deeply focused contemplation of the students; the relationship between student and object is palpable. This is particularly striking in the drawing "Hand holding skeleton hand" by Amy Ou (page 67). The student places her left hand over the skeleton of a left hand, and then draws both with her right. It is an image both intimate and unsettling.

Art & Anatomy also allows students to contemplate the emotional resonance of what they are experiencing. As student Karen M. Ong noted, "I had never before confronted death in any significant way," (p. 107) a sentiment likely common to the vast majority of first-year medical students. Anatomy lab can be a particularly overwhelming way of meeting death for the first time. Approaching it through drawing—focusing on a single bone, or one particular organ—can offer a more accessible entrée. The very specificity of this experience encourages more nuance: considerations of beauty as well as grief, reflection as well as education, form as well as function.

One of the more chilling moments in the standard cadaver dissection is the bisection of the head. After the brain has been removed, students use a power saw to slice the remainder of the head in half, with a clean slice down the middle. This renders clear an otherwise incomprehensible anatomy of the

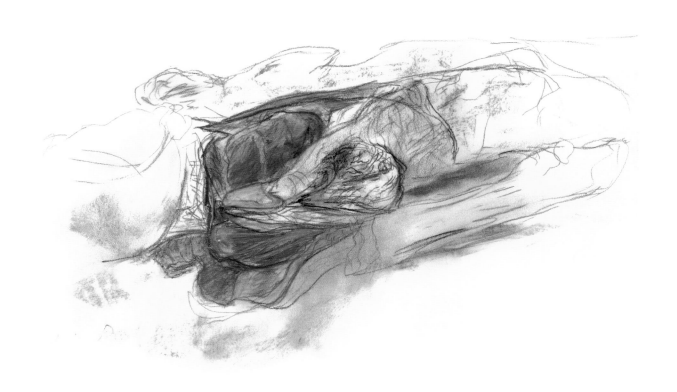

Karen M. Ong, Cadaver ("Under My Skin")

head. For my dissection team, this was a chasm that stopped us dead in our tracks. Cutting open the breastbone and mucking around in the thorax was one thing; cutting through the head was orders of magnitude more terrifying. We'd kept the face of our cadaver covered until that point. But now we had to face her humanity and also violate it.

Drawing straws, it fell to me to wield the saw. As I powered it through the layers of bone and muscle, gritting my teeth and my emotions, I thought about the dissectors of yore. I thought about Vesalius and Leonardo, who had undertaken these very same cuts centuries earlier, albeit with cruder tools. I wondered how they navigated the fraught negotiations of humanity versus inquiry. It is an incongruity that every medical practitioner must wrestle with.

Michael Malone's "Bisected Head" (p. 115) confronts this paradox directly. The left side of the head is the cadaver's face in its untouched state. The right side of the head depicts the fully bisected and dissected head. Yet the two parts are drawn nearly connected, so that the head almost feels both whole and dissected at the same time. The face of the woman and the underlying structures that create that face—as well as the cutting the student has done to reveal those structures—are able to be joined together in a way that would be difficult in real life. The artistic rendering enables us to appreciate the emotional grappling one must do in the world of anatomy and in the larger world of medicine.

The "art of medicine" is a term that is used—sometimes disparagingly—to refer to the non-technical skills of medicine. Certainly Vesalius and Leonardo amply demonstrated that the art of medicine can be extremely rigorous even while being remarkably aesthetic. The students who spent these additional hours in Art & Anatomy had the benefit of being steeped in the literal art of medicine. Readers of this illuminating book will have that chance too.

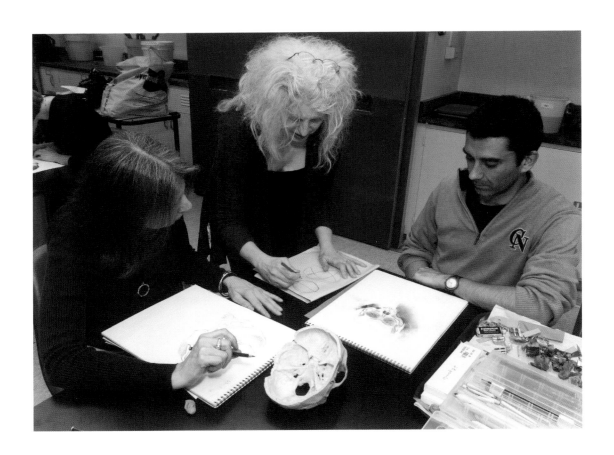

Learning to See: Anatomy Through Artists' Eyes

An Introduction from Artist in Residence Laura Ferguson

On Tuesday evenings at the NYU School of Medicine, art supplies are set out on tables and the Anatomy Lab is transformed into a studio, with a great spirit of creative enterprise. The drawings made here – by med students, doctors, and other medical professionals – show how powerful and compelling the imagery of anatomy can be. They invite us not just inside the body, but into the rite of passage that is gross anatomy.

This is Art & Anatomy, a unique drawing seminar in NYUSoM's Master Scholars Program in Humanistic Medicine. The program is part of a growing movement in medicine that encourages a more empathetic attitude toward patients and recognizes the value of listening to their voices, especially through the expressive power of the arts.

I created Art & Anatomy in 2009, as part of an artist residency at the medical school. The idea came out of my own work as an artist, the many years I spent exploring my own anatomy and finding beauty in a curving spine. I came to my role with a strong personal investment in using art to influence a new generation of more empathetic medical professionals. In making my own drawings, I had come to see my spine as a graceful curve, suggesting flow and movement, with a subtle balance arising out of asymmetry. But the medical world did not seem open to an aesthetic that saw spinal curves – or any unusual anatomies – as graceful, and I hoped to play a role in changing those perceptions. I knew the transformative power of art would help students engage with the emotional challenges of the dissection experience, and in a creative space where expressiveness and openness are valued, allow them to see past death and discover the beauty of the living human body.

Our intent: learning to see

There's nothing like drawing something for really learning about it; you spend so much time communing with your subject, you come to know it in a deep way. It becomes part of the body's memory.

I knew that drawing was a great way to learn anatomy. Holding the drawing class in the Anatomy Lab grounds humanism in a rigorous learning process directly related to medical knowledge and professional skill. Here med students sit side by side with faculty and staff, and beginners with more accomplished artists. The surprising number who have come to medical school from an arts or humanities background find a place to integrate their dual loves for art and science.

Drawing is a process of discovery and learning – a kind of quest. In Art & Anatomy, we value process more than end results; even if we don't make great drawings, the process will bring us a deeper knowledge of anatomy. Our goal is not making masterpieces, but learning to see.

The key to good drawing lies in letting go of preconceptions and learning to see what's really there. This openness takes us away from value judgments like good/bad, beautiful/ugly, healthy/sick. Art allows many different realities to be present together, without the need to draw conclusions or make choices. It brings us into a state of mindfulness, where we're fully engaged, curious and motivated to learn, making connections, and on the deepest level, connecting with the creativity of the body.

A large bulletin board in the Anatomy Lab is filled with drawings made in Art & Anatomy, and many visitors spend time admiring the art. But recently I overheard the comment that our work didn't measure up to that of famous medical illustrator Frank Netter, and it occurred to me that I should make clear our very different intent. In Art & Anatomy we're not trying to match the detail and accuracy of a Netter, or make textbook illustrations of the most typical, most "normal" version of each anatomical structure. Rather, our goal is to learn, and to share with our friends and families and fellow students what we've learned, about the beauty of anatomy and the part it plays in our lives. We don't always have the tools or technique to get what we've seen onto the paper, to allow others to see through our eyes, but that is the goal: to bring others into the experience … and to remind ourselves, later, of what we saw, how we felt about it, where we were at this moment in our learning process and in our lives. The expressiveness of drawing means that we're conveying a lot of this in our work whether we try to or not. If we can just be in the moment, enter into the experience, a lot will – and does – come across.

Insight into the dissection experience

I'm a great believer in the power of art – to express things that can't be as easily communicated in other ways – and to share experiences that go deep into the human spirit and psyche – the same places where illness or pain often take us. Art engenders empathy and human connection between artist and viewer: an imaginative entering into the consciousness of another.

Art goes deep and so does the Anatomy Lab experience. The dissection of a cadaver evokes complex emotional responses for medical students, due to its inescapable confrontation with death and the visceral reality of the body.

Although we can only see inside the body after death, our anatomies are central to our every experience as living, breathing, moving human beings. Dissection is the closest we can come to seeing inside the living body, and to me, the Anatomy Lab represents true humanism: an incredible opportunity to see a great variety of real human bodies, donated for us to learn from. Like drawing, dissection is hands-on, tactile and visual. But the imagery of anatomy has become so associated with the medical – and thus with pathology, disease, and death – that it has lost its associations with the living body. We don't have many beautiful images to relate to when we think of our inner bodies, and that has contributed to making us squeamish and even fearful of visualizing them.

Students come to the Anatomy Lab with great curiosity, but often with that same discomfort about what they may have to confront. They may hesitate to show their emotions. Should they be stoical and emotionally neutral? or sensitive and empathetic? They're probably feeling both.

Because it requires cutting a human body – something that would in other circumstances be "judged a desecration," in the words of poet-physician Jack Coulehan – dissection is an emotionally complicated task. Christine Montross, who wrote about her own dissection experience in *Body of Work*, describes how after getting used to doing brutal, hurtful things to the cadaver, it becomes easier to do them to patients. She quotes 18th century surgeon and anatomist William Hunter, who memorably wrote that Anatomy "familiarizes the heart to a kind of necessary IN-humanity."

Medical students often regard cadavers as their "first patients," and dissection is their first experience of "hurting to heal" – though, as I discovered during my childhood scoliosis surgery, the necessity for "hurting" is usually not acknowledged. But it causes discomfort all the same – like all unacknowledged things.

So it's not surprising that for many students, their time in the cadaver lab begins a process of emotional detachment. Since drawing is not invasive, and involves only looking, it can help them to have a more engaged and positive experience of the Anatomy Lab. Because it's inherently expressive, drawing offers students a way to process their feelings and reconnect with the humanity of the bodies they're privileged to learn from.

In Art & Anatomy, I've tried to create an environment that's open and accepting of whatever feelings they do choose to express. I let the atmosphere of a studio, and the knowledge that we're there to make art, evoke a certain depth and meaningfulness. Students may be reluctant to talk about their feelings, or unaware of them, but they can still express them in the process of drawing, without needing words – and they may feel better afterwards, without knowing why.

When I'm helping students to decide what to draw, or to understand what they're looking at, I point out details of the bones or cadavers – but my purpose is not so much to teach them anatomy as to call their attention to beauty. Seeing anatomy as beautiful can be profound. If you can see beauty, and find a way to show it in a drawing, it can make you feel better about the whole experience – about yourself and your ability to cope. You're doing something good for this person whose body you also have to cut: seeing them, and giving them respect and appreciation. This makes it easier to stay engaged. There's a big payoff in staying open to the full range of your feelings and responses.

A portrait comes alive through an artist's ability to evoke the individual, and in Art & Anatomy we learn to appreciate the uniqueness of each body's inner space. Bones are wonderful and endlessly challenging to draw: curved and subtly spiraled to enhance their options for movement, with surfaces marked by the pull of muscles, creating movement throughout the person's life. Each bone is unique – and their details tell the story of a life lived.

This offers a way in to anatomy that's more personal, less generic – that sees and values individuality. Here we don't need to learn about or recognize pathologies; instead we can focus on beauty. These artists are imagining the living body as they draw: looking at bones and cadavers but imagining the person who once inhabited them – and also imagining the living, moving anatomy within themselves. Looking at their drawings, viewers can share this experience and inhabit their own anatomies more fully.

A new art of anatomy

Art looks beneath the surface of life – but strangely enough, it rarely looks beneath the surface of the skin. For Leonardo da Vinci, drawing anatomy was an essential part of his artistic investigations into the nature of human experience. But 500 years later, he is still the one great artist of anatomy who comes to mind. Though artists traditionally study anatomy as an aid to drawing the figure, anatomical art became sidelined into the genre of medical illustration. Those scientifically accurate images are valuable, but should they be the only images we have? Does the imagery of anatomy belong solely to the world of medicine? How do we relate to our inner bodies if we imagine them as textbook illustrations: generic, one-size-fits-all, and diagrammatic, with the texture of real life smoothed away?

When I first looked for images of my own curving spine, the only ones I found showed scoliosis at its most unattractive: a figure awkwardly bending forward, appearing exaggeratedly hunchbacked. Those of us with unusual anatomies feel an implied judgment when our differences are seen that way: it's an aesthetic of ugliness that equates to defectiveness. Art offers an alternative aesthetic, one where every body can have its own beauty, grace, originality, or allure.

Our inner landscapes are unique, visually interesting, even beautiful, full of complex spatial configurations, and grounded in the texture and detail of physical reality. Art can show us this beauty and endow it with meaning and insight; it can capture the uniqueness of our inner bodies and help us to connect with them more closely. We need art that takes anatomy out of the realm of the medical and returns it to the personal.

A drawing is like a handwritten letter from artist to viewer – handmade, imperfect, and by its very nature more human, more relatable – and better at communicating the texture of reality. These Art & Anatomy drawings come out of a medical school and were made by medical students and professionals – but their intent is not medical, it's simply human. They make manifest the power of art to communicate in unique ways that words sometimes cannot – and in the pages that follow, they will speak for themselves. I hope they speak to you.

About the Master Scholars Program in Humanistic Medicine

by Katie Grogan, DMH, MA, Associate Director

For nearly twenty years, the Master Scholars Program in Humanistic Medicine (MSPHM) has been advancing interdisciplinary and interprofessional education at NYU School of Medicine. The MSPHM develops elective, non-credit seminars in medical humanities, designed to cultivate creative and intellectual interests typically underrepresented in medical education and culture. These seminars engage medicine in dialogue with history, literature, philosophy, ethics, creative writing, and visual arts. They push the limits of the biomedical model and explore other frameworks for understanding health, illness, and the human condition.

Art & Anatomy has been a core component of the MSPHM since Laura Ferguson first created the seminar in 2009. It is offered every fall and spring and has had approximately 400 participants to date. Students can enroll at any point, though many opt to do so concurrently with their various anatomy modules during the first eighteen months of medical school, or multiple times across all four years. Like all endeavors of the MSPHM, Art & Anatomy is intended for medical students but open to all members of the NYU School of Medicine community. This unique format enables the seminar to traverse the boundaries between art and science but also between professional hierarchies. Students, faculty, and staff sit alongside one another, learning to transform anatomy into art. This is one of the crucial contributions of arts-based pedagogies in medicine: the reduction, or even erasure, of the entrenched power differentials characteristic of the medical profession.[1]

The arts and humanities celebrate fluidity and diversity of expression, while challenging binary thinking and the imperative of a single correct interpretation. Art & Anatomy trains participants to see the human body with an artist's eye, complementing or contrasting that view with the lenses through which they may typically see it—those of student, clinician, or researcher, for instance. The Anatomy Lab becomes a space for both scientific inquiry and creative expression; cadavers can be both grotesque and beautiful; they can be something in between person and object; we can be simultaneously repelled and drawn in; being there can feel like an act of intrusion and one of reverence. Art & Anatomy epitomizes the mission of the MSPHM to deepen learners' reflective capacity and enhance their tolerance for ambiguity, in the lab and beyond.

1 Haidet P et al. 2016. A guiding framework to maximize the power of the arts in medical education: a systematic review and metasynthesis. Medical Education 50: 320-331. doi:10.1111/medu.12925

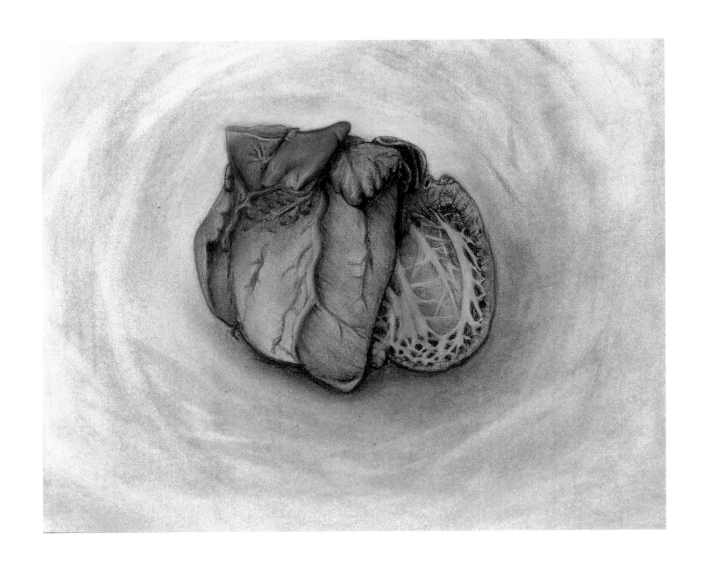

Hannah Bernstein, Heart ("Open Heart")

Art & Anatomy: A Student Perspective

Hannah Bernstein, MD/PhD Candidate, Class of 2020

Science and art have always been my two greatest passions, and my favorite subject in both cases is people. Art & Anatomy combines all of these themes, which is why I was so drawn to this course offered through the Master Scholars Program in Humanistic Medicine. I'm so glad I followed my instincts, because it has been one of the most rewarding and valuable parts of my medical education so far.

In medical school, you're constantly bombarded with information in the form of lectures and textbooks about human anatomy and physiology. It can be overwhelming, and in order to simplify it all I found myself relying on an abstract and idealized version of how the human body works. It wasn't until I started anatomy lab that I was forced out of the textbooks and exposed for the first time to real examples of human anatomy. Being a visual learner, the ability to see and hold actual flesh and bones made all those facts I had learned real for me. Undoubtedly, holding a human heart and dissecting out the coronary arteries is an irreplaceable experience; and yet for me there was still something missing. The goal of anatomy lab is to teach anatomy, which it does very well; but trying to learn all the muscles, nerves, blood vessels, and bones of the arm in a week or two doesn't give you much time to really appreciate what you're seeing.

That's what Art & Anatomy did for me. It made me look at the body with the eye of an artist, and I was blown away by the complexity, elegance, and even beauty of the bones and organs that I saw when I changed my perspective. Laura showed us how to see the inherent beauty in bodies of all shapes and sizes, to focus on the incredible details and appreciate the amount of variation that exists in all of us. When I created drawings for the course I tried to capture this appreciation for the beauty and variation of the human body. I learned to appreciate things that aren't conventionally beautiful, like the curves of the femur and the intricate network of blood vessels covering the heart. I also learned that in general, real people don't look like textbook illustrations. No two people are the same, and no one is "perfect." Each body has its own unique deviations, and this applies to what's inside as much as what's on the surface. This is an important lesson for any future doctor, and I'm grateful that I got to learn it from such a unique perspective.

There is also something cathartic about drawing. No matter how busy or stressed out I was during the first part of medical school, I could show up at the anatomy lab and just draw for an hour and a half, and let everything else go. I got to be creative, and experiment with technique, and create something beautiful. Drawing helped keep me sane, and put the rest of medical school in perspective. I feel so lucky that I got to participate in such a unique and fulfilling class, and I know that it was an experience I won't ever forget.

"It was a delight that the School of Medicine would make such a course available to the students and faculty. The notion of 'slowing down' and taking the time to pursue other than medicine/science activities is important to the well-being of students and faculty alike."

– Harold Horowitz, MD, Professor, Division of Infectious Diseases and Immunology

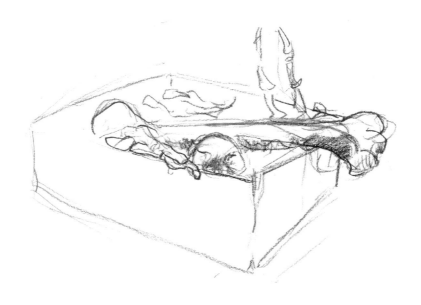

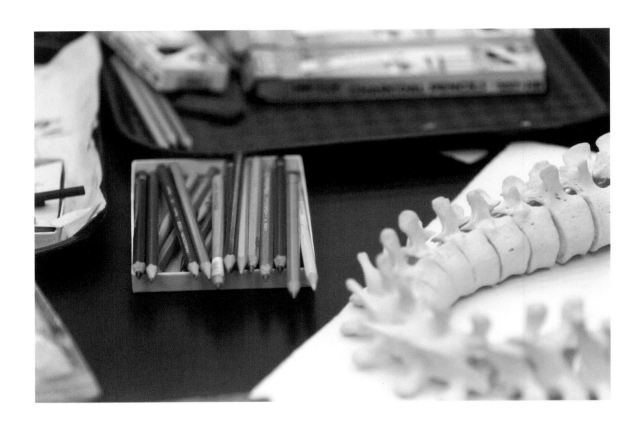

We meet in the Anatomy Lab, transformed on Tuesday evenings
into a studio. Art supplies are provided: graphite, pastel and color pencils; charcoal,
Conté crayons, and felt-tip markers; and a drawing pad for each student.

On tables in the study room, some students work on drawings of bones; in the
dissection rooms, others set up easels and draw from the cadavers.

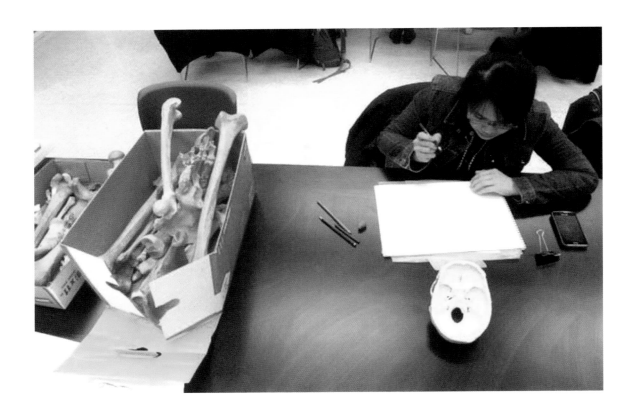

Each student chooses a bone to draw, and we begin.

The hours of drawing bring a state of deep focus and concentration – an experience of mindfulness, of being present in the moment. We learn to let go of preconceptions and be open to what we're seeing. Making each drawing becomes a process of discovery and learning that takes students inside their own bodies and changes their relationship to the space within.

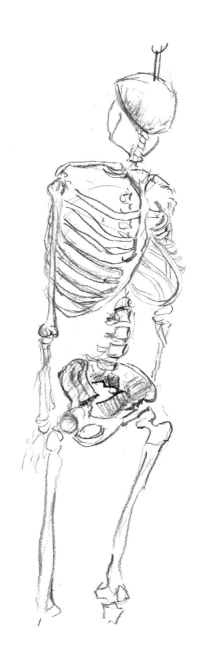

Harold Horowitz, Hanging skeleton

ART & ANATOMY:
DRAWINGS

The drawings that follow are loosely grouped by region of the body.
Captions give the artist's name and a simple description of the anatomical
subject matter. Titles given by the artists, if any, are shown in parentheses.

A complete list of artists and artworks, with page numbers, appears at the
back of the book.

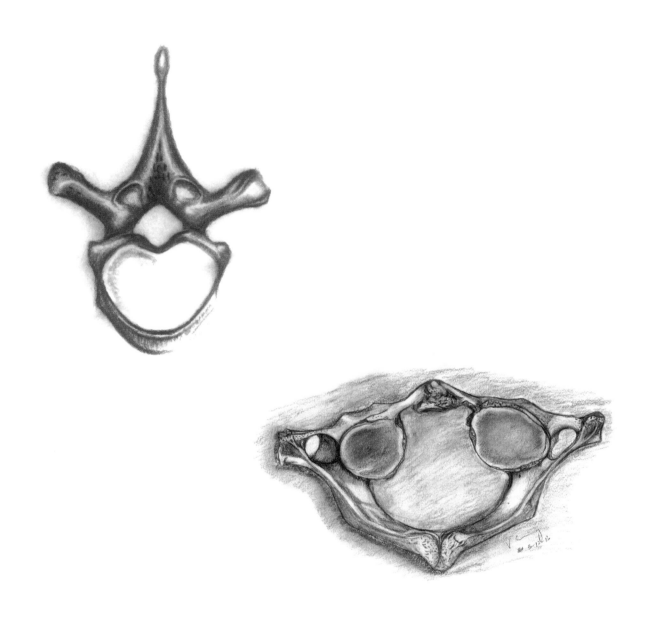

above: Kathy May Tran, Vertebra (thoracic) | below: Vicky Chiang, Vertebra (cervical)

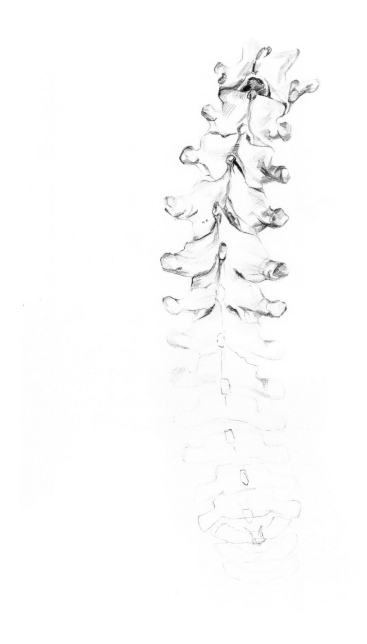

Emma Trawick, Vertebral column

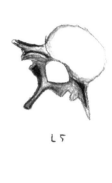

L5

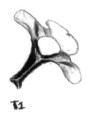

T1

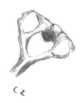

C2

Coccyx1

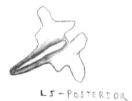

L5-POSTERIOR

2013 GHC

Gabriel Campion, 6 Vertebrae

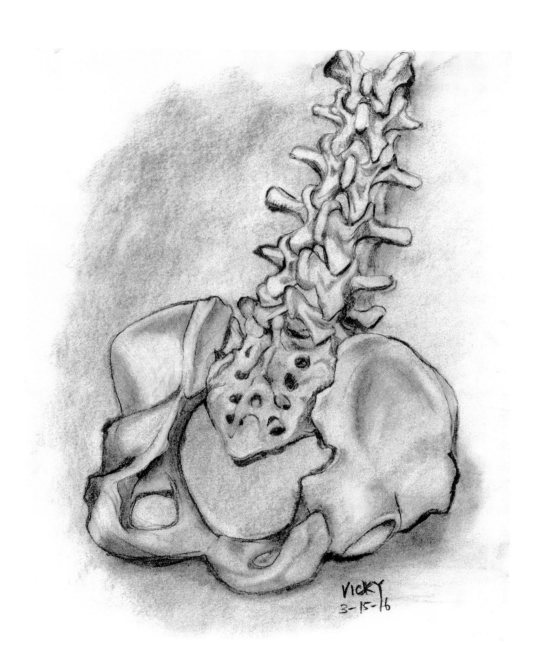

Vicky Chiang, Lumbar spine with sacrum and pelvis

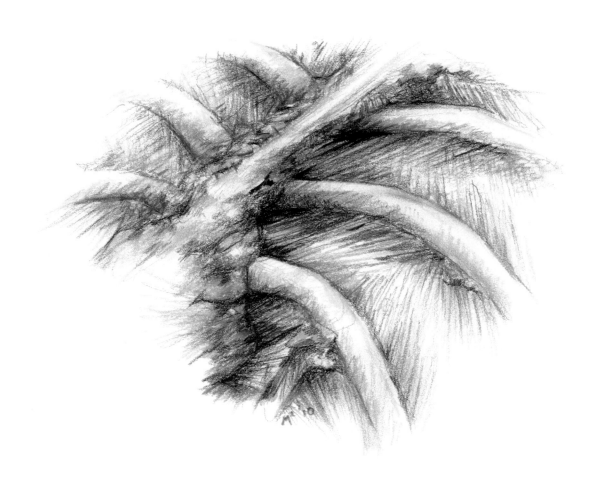

Michael Malone, Ribs with intercostal muscles ("Deforestation")

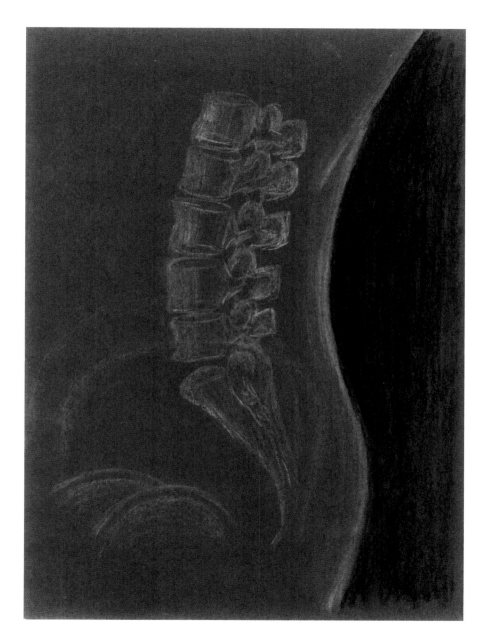

Shian Liu, Lumbar spine and sacrum (from x-ray)

"I unexpectedly gained friends through the seminar. The anatomy lab brings so many different kinds of people together – scientists, professional artists, medical students, pre-medical students, teachers, former doctors, current doctors, photographers, spine surgeons – and reminds us that our physical bodies exist in a wonderful tension between uniformity and uniqueness."

– Shian Liu, MD, class of 2015

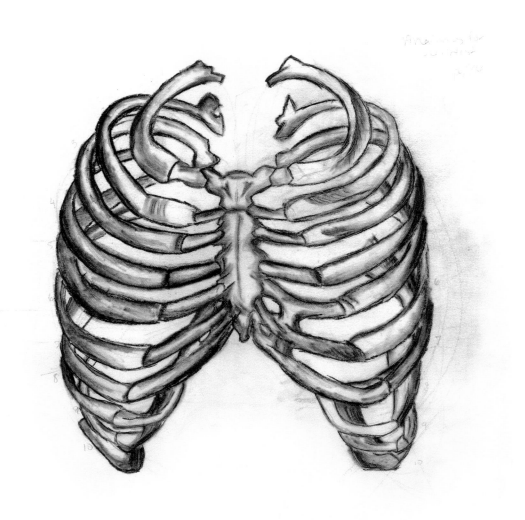

Shian Liu, Ribcage ("Ribcage, of Breath and Bone")

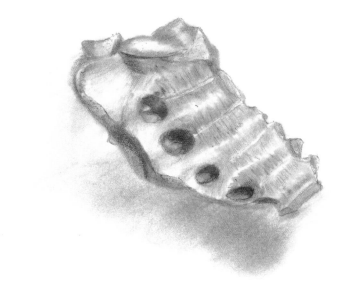

Arielle Haves Bayer, Sacrum

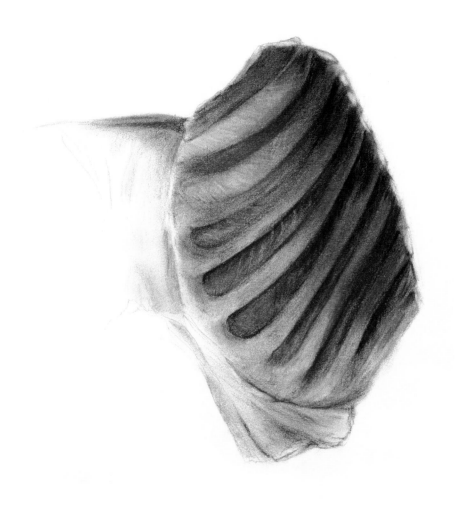

Silvia Curado, Ribs with light shining through

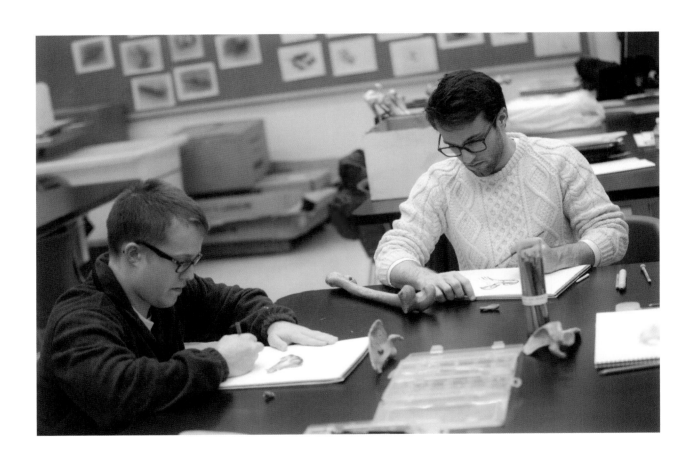

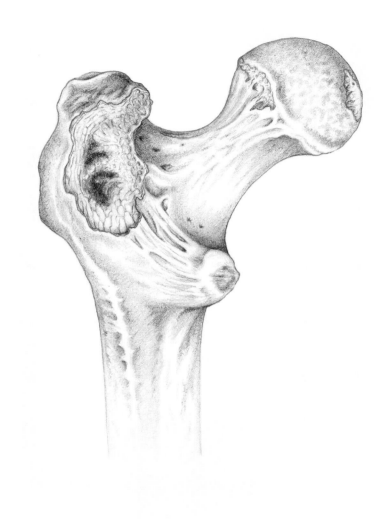

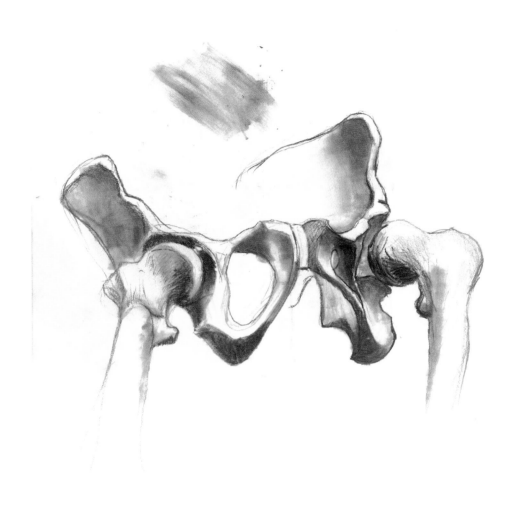

David Fooksman, Pelvis with hip joints

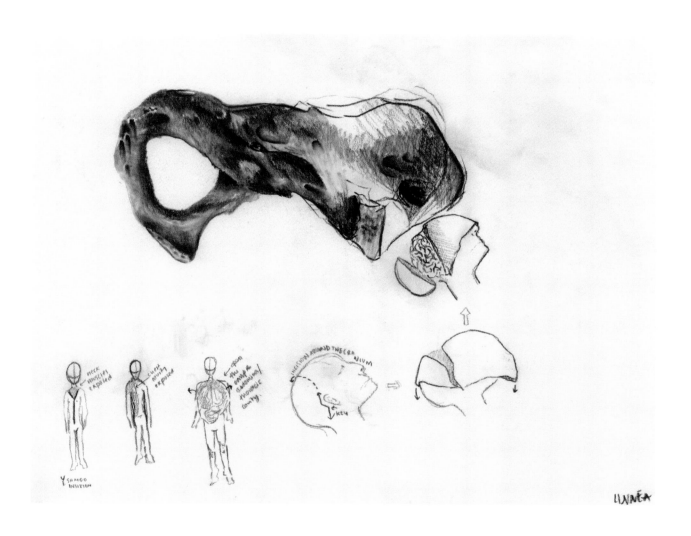

Linnea Russell, Pelvis with sketches

"The experience has made me more appreciative of the aesthetics and strength of the human body. Even after death, the spirit of the bodies live on in art. I hoped to capture the life of the human skeletal system using imaginative positioning of the pieces. Thank you for giving me the opportunity to explore the beauty of the body's natural tapestry."

– Jing Ye, class of 2018

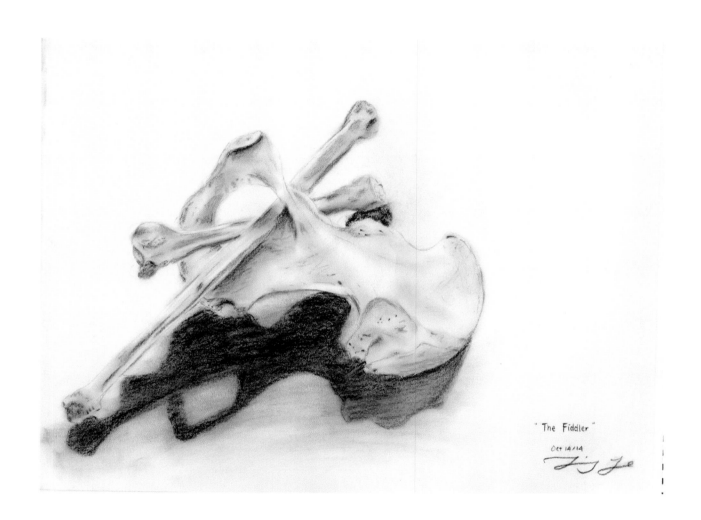

"The Fiddler"

Oct 14/14

Jing Ye, Pelvis with fibula and radius ("The Fiddler")

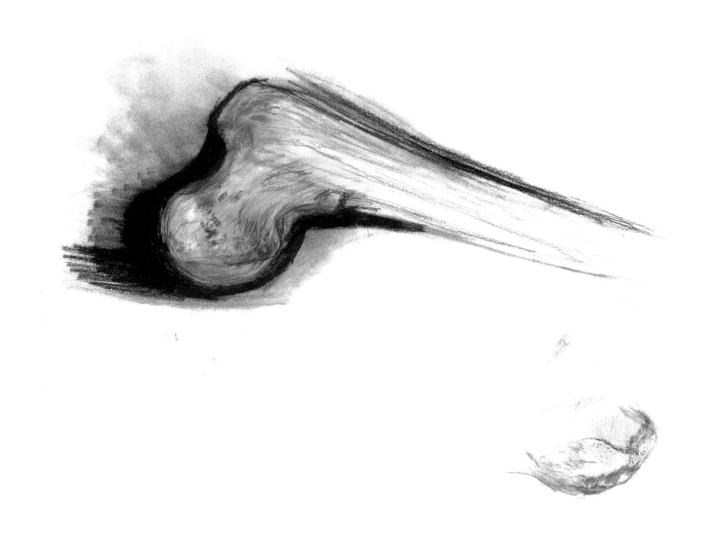

Alejandra Yancey, Femur studies

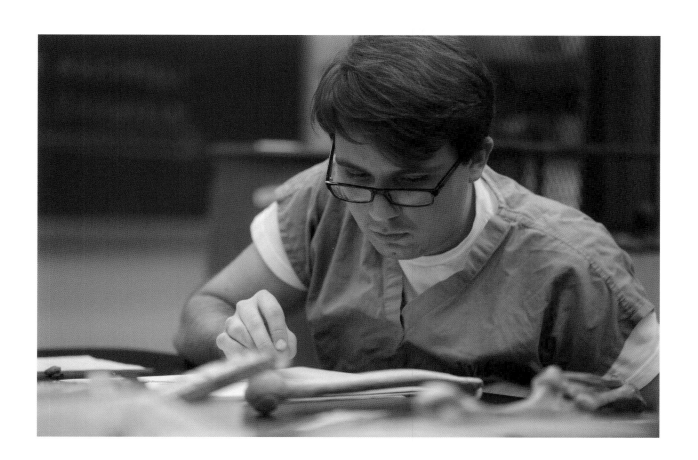

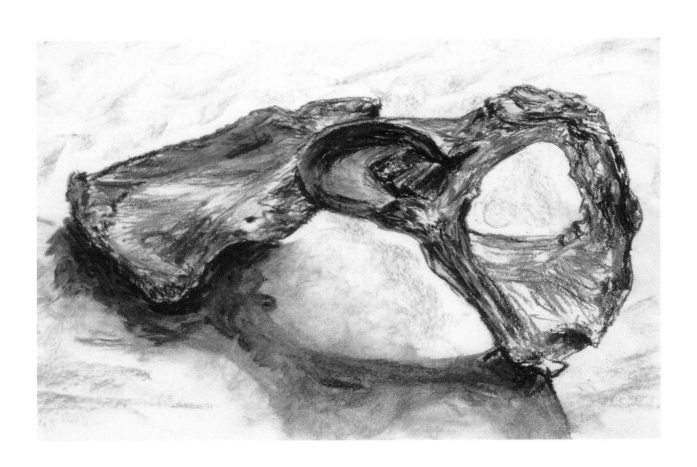

Julia Goldberg, Pelvis

46

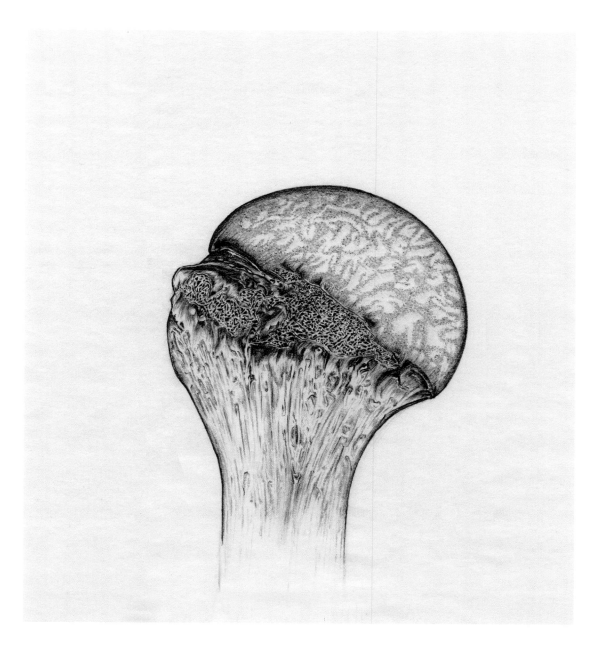

Kevin Efros, Head of femur

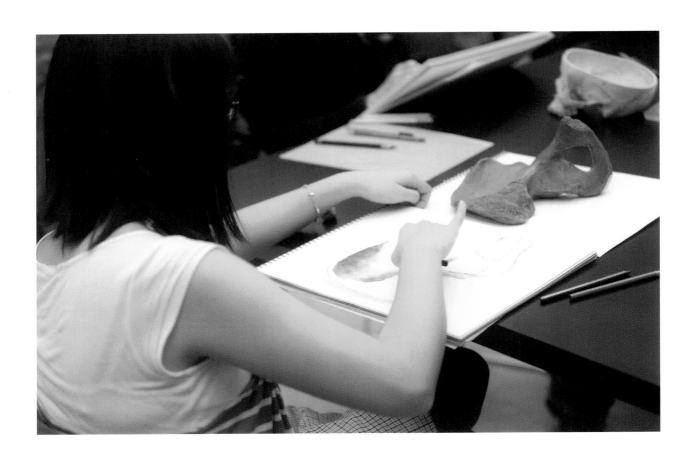

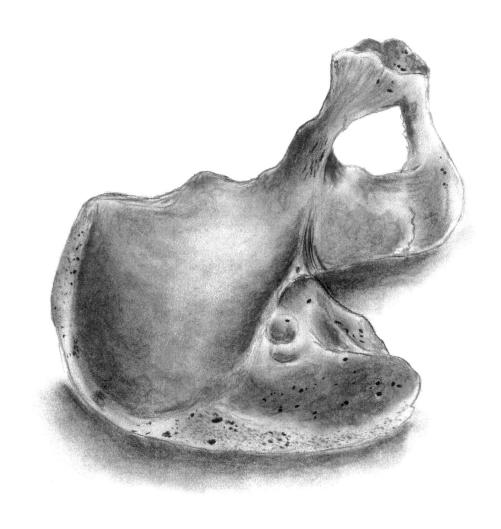

Susanna Nguy, Pelvis ("Hip Hip")

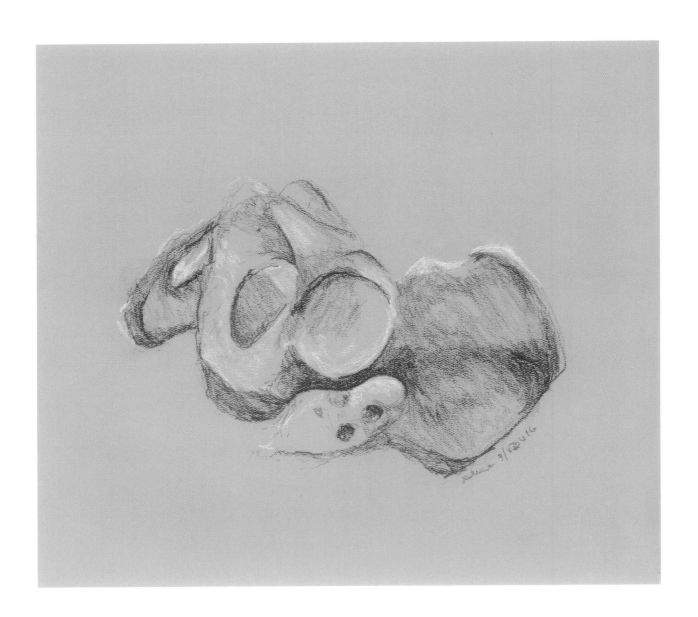

Arlene Paul, Pelvis

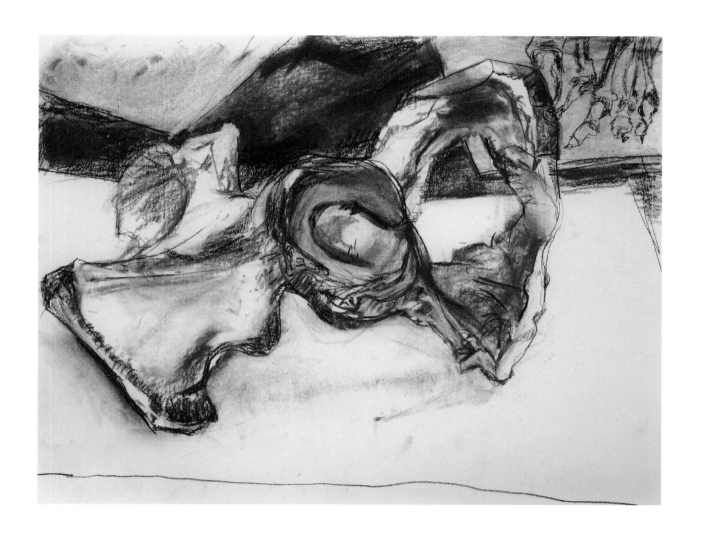

Michael Cammer, Pelvis study

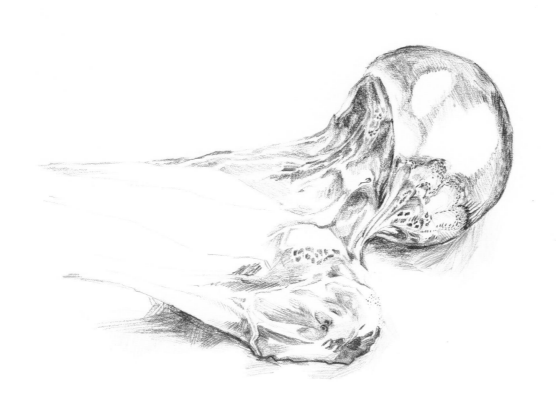

Emma Trawick, Head of femur

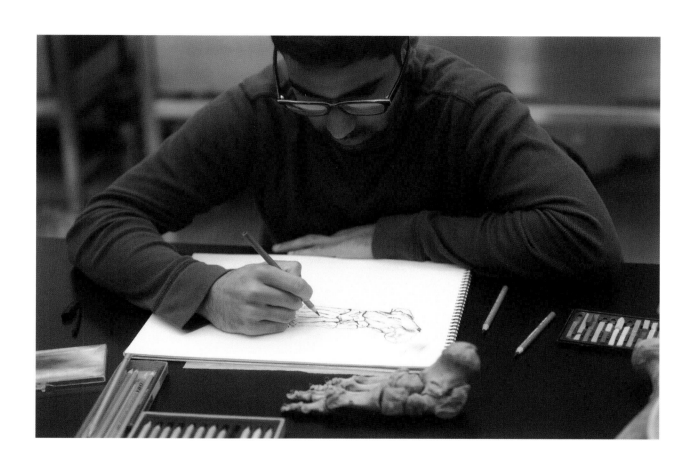

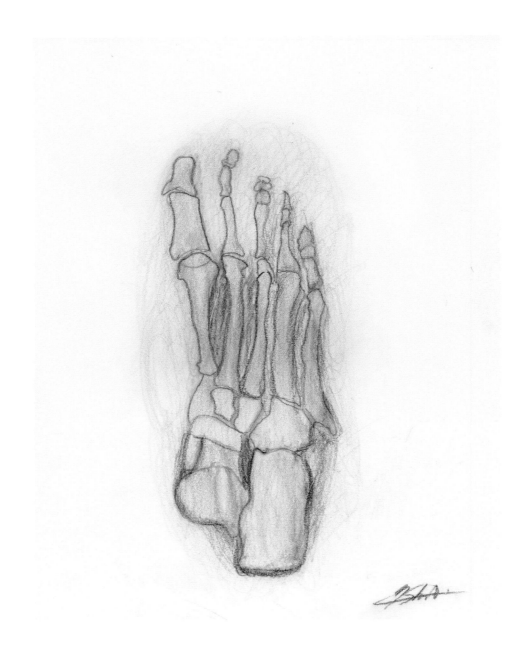

Nihar P. Shah, Skeleton foot

54

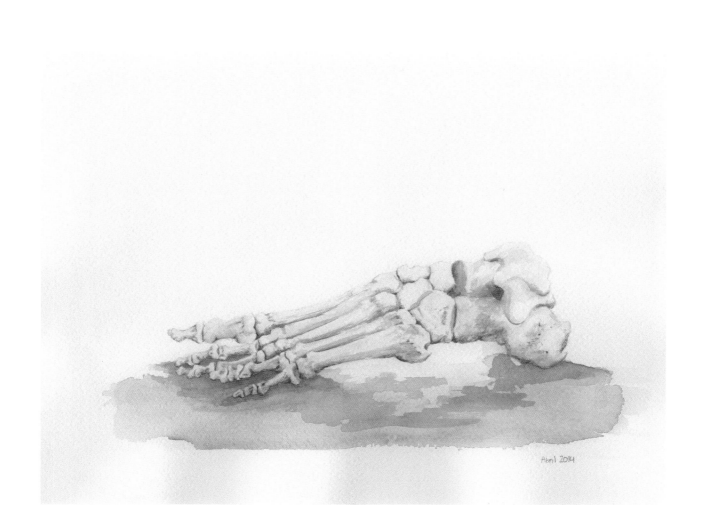

Valeria Mezzano, Foot

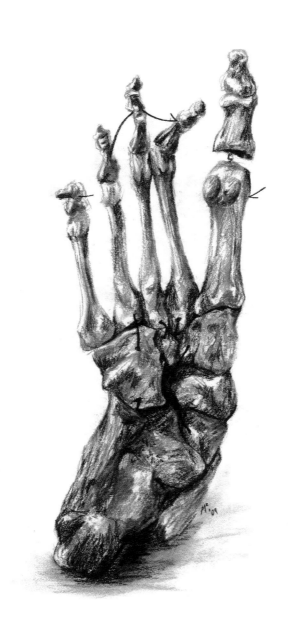

Michael Malone, Skeleton foot ("Monument")

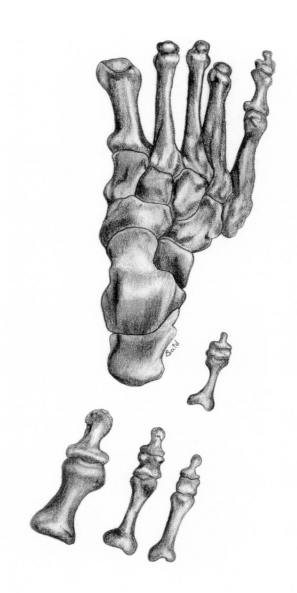

Said S. Saab, Skeleton foot with toes (after Albinus/Wandelaar)

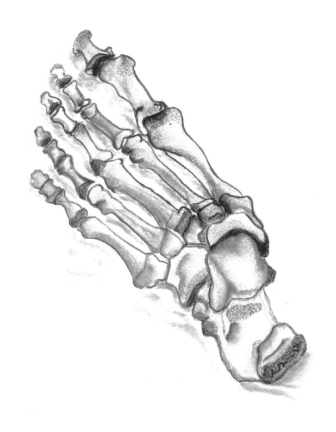

Alejandro Gomez-Viso, Skeleton foot

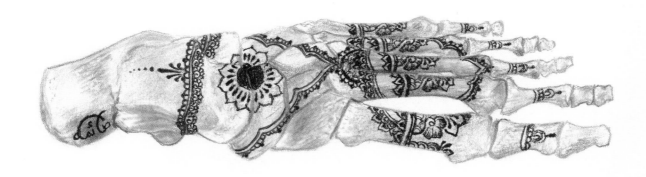

Saima Usmani, Skeleton foot ("Has Anybody Seen the Bride's Foot?")

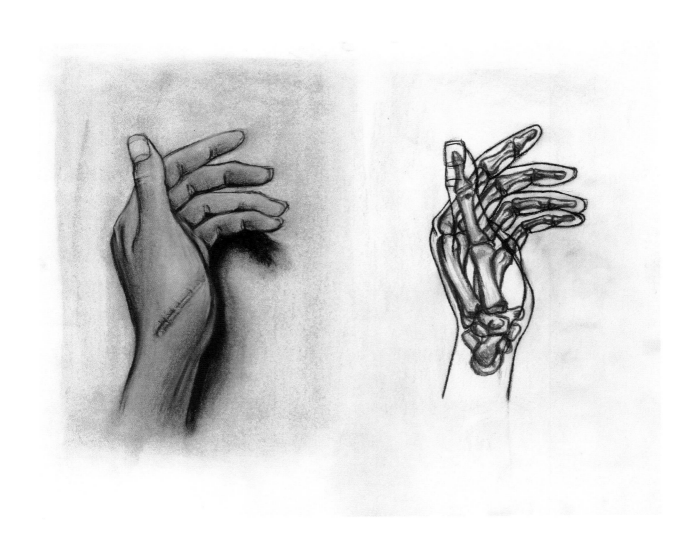

Hannah Bernstein, Double hands ("Hand with a Scar")

We draw our own hands, feeling and visualizing the bones, muscles, and tendons just under the surface.

Our own individual differences – a scar, a broken finger – help to connect us to the individuality of each anatomical structure.

"As a neurotic medical student with no art experience, I remember feeling anxious about whether or not I would be skilled at drawing. That feeling quickly changed, however, when I finished my first drawing and looked down at the sketch with a great sense of satisfaction. The connection I felt to my profession was overwhelming. As the weeks progressed, I sketched various bones of the body as physicians and anatomists throughout history had done before me. Each session became an escape from the rigors of medical school where I took an hour to reflect on the subject I love."

– Matthew Pergamo, MD, class of 2017

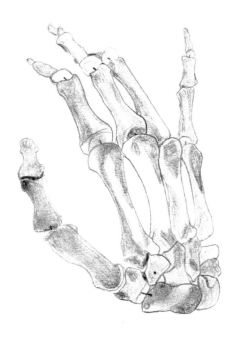

Matthew Pergamo, Hand skeleton ("From Novice to Old Hand")

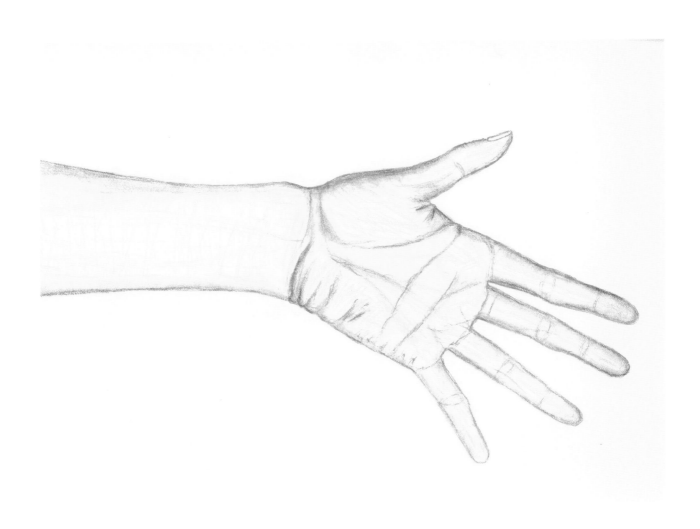

Lizbeth Hu, Hand ("Handy 201")

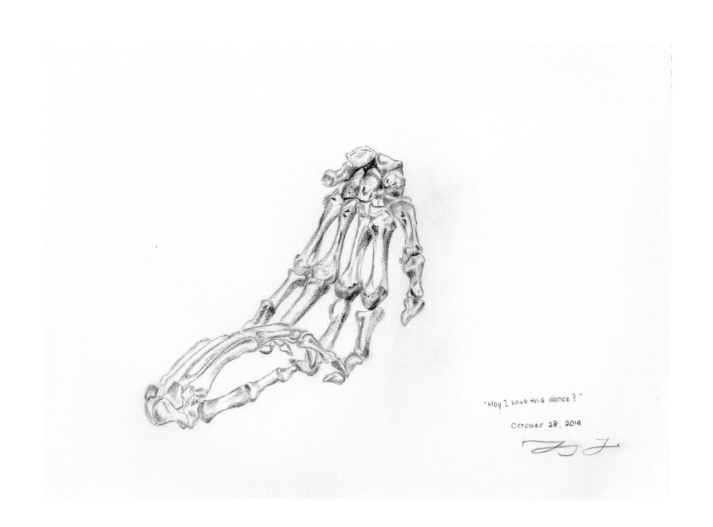

"May I have this dance?"

October 28, 2014

Jing Ye, Linked hands ("May I Have This Dance?")

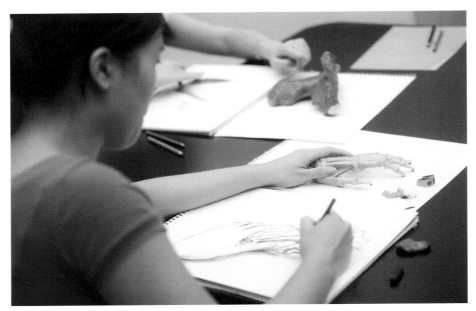

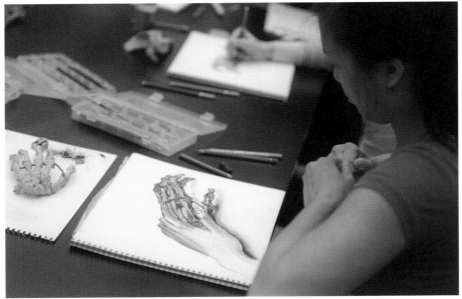

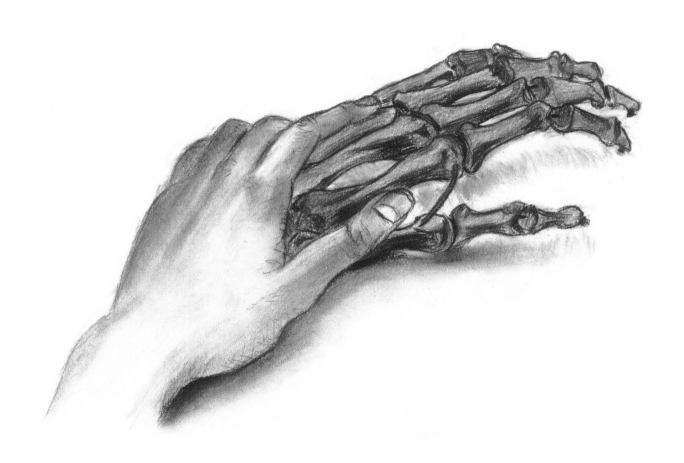

Amy Ou, Hand holding skeleton hand

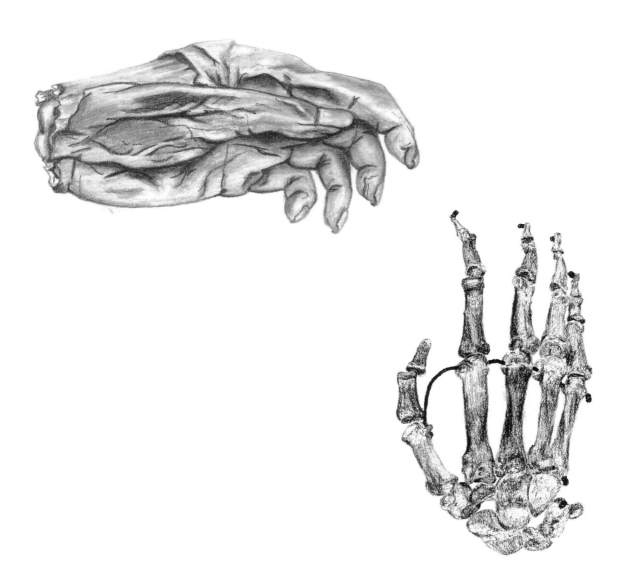

above: Jessica Meyer, Cadaver hand ("Work for Idle Hands")
below: Clarissa Lam, Hand skeleton

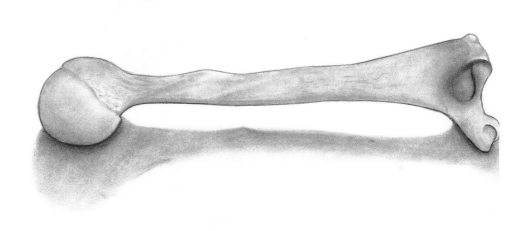

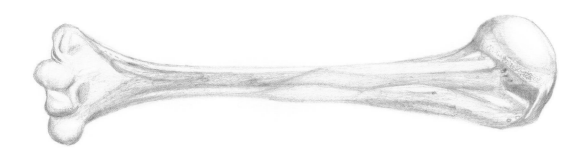

above: Ariana Ilene Rabinowitsch, Humerus ("Long Bone") | below: Andrew C. Lin, Humerus ("Stability")

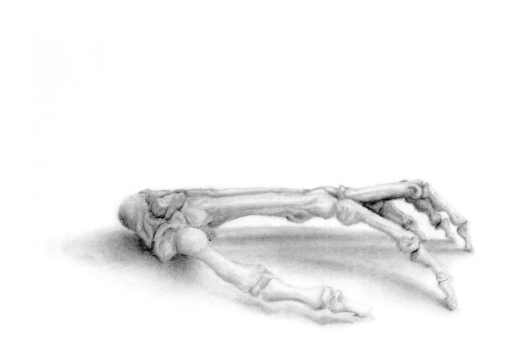

Kyle Anthony Durrant, Skeleton hand ("The Hand")

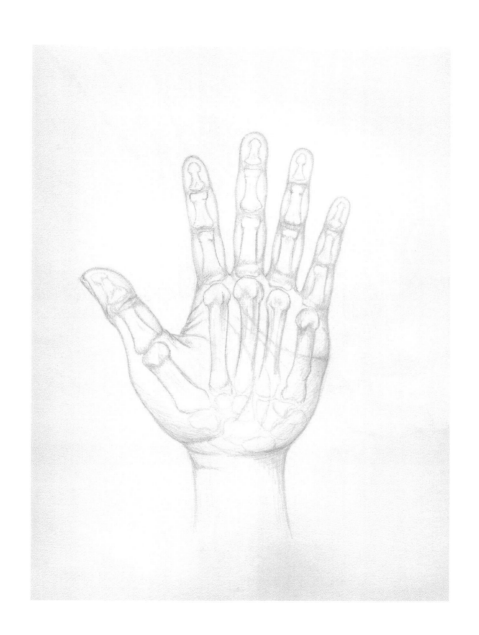

Lindy Triebes, Hand with hand skeleton

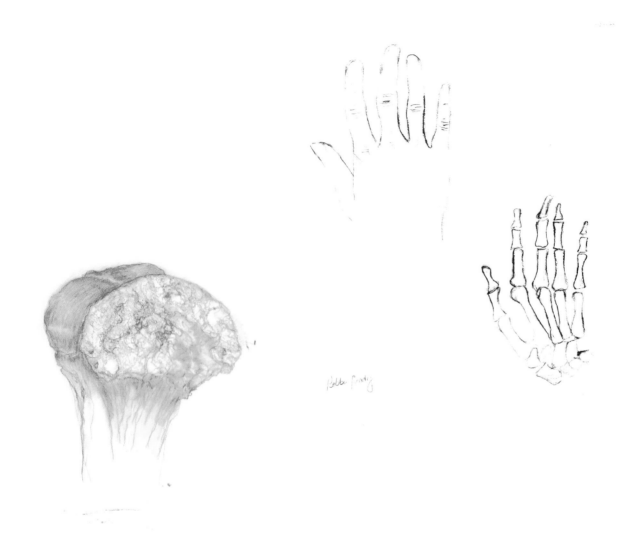

left: Wendy Agudo, Humerus ("Mechanics of the Body") | right: Bobbi Georgia Brady, Hand skeleton ("Handy Imperfection")

"Variation in human anatomy is like a small window into that person's life. It is the variation that we learn from; the subtlety of a normal variant from a pathologic variant is often what differentiates a good doctor from a great doctor. The intimacy of drawing these subtleties while training to become a doctor is somehow a humble experience, but yet also very profound."

– Bobbi Georgia Brady, MD, class of 2014

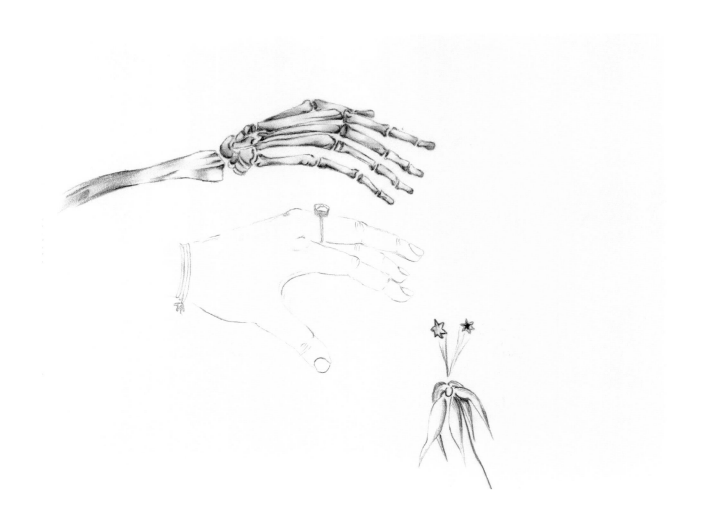

Kella L. Vangsness, Hand with hand skeleton

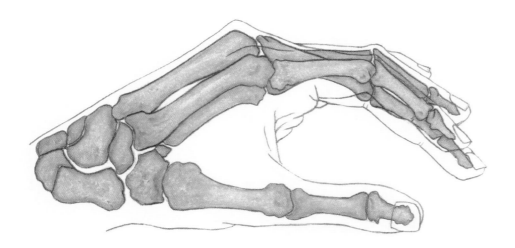

Kyra Doumlele, Hand with skeleton

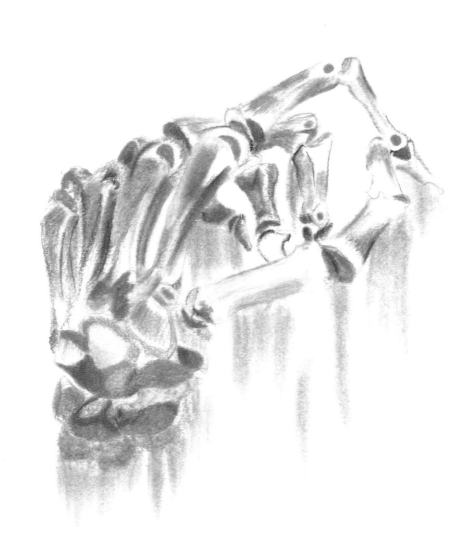

Annie Wang, Hand skeleton ("Heavy-handed")

"Art & Anatomy was a wonderful course that taught me to appreciate the form of various parts of the body. I learned to focus on the intricate details in the context of the overall structures."

– Annie Wang, MD, class of 2016

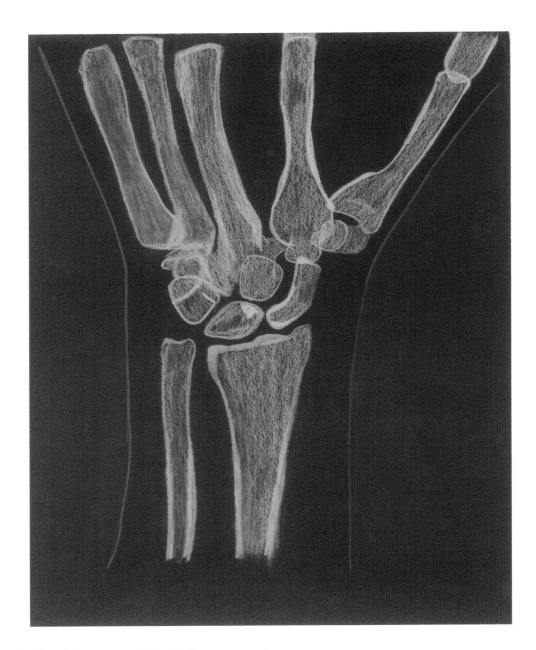

Sarah Azarchi, Hand, from x-ray ("Wrist Fluoroscopy")

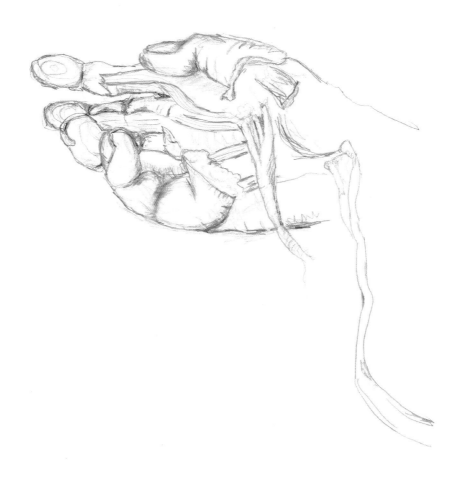

Samuel M. Cohen, Hand with tendons

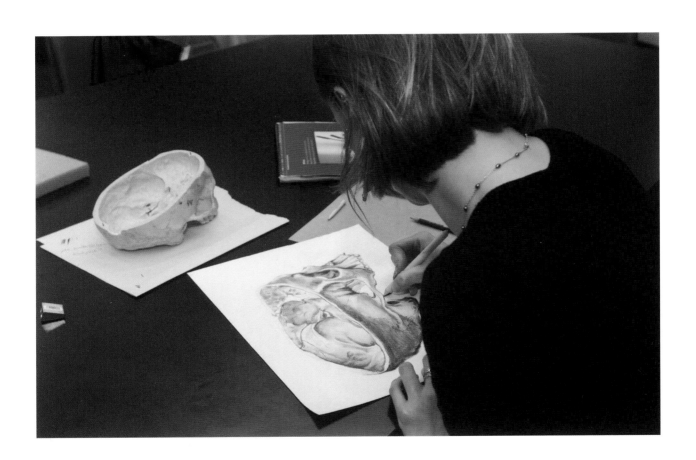

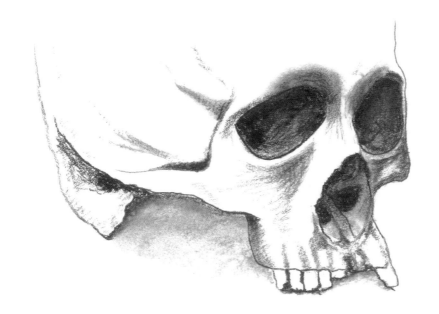

Milesh Patel

Milesh Patel, Skull

81

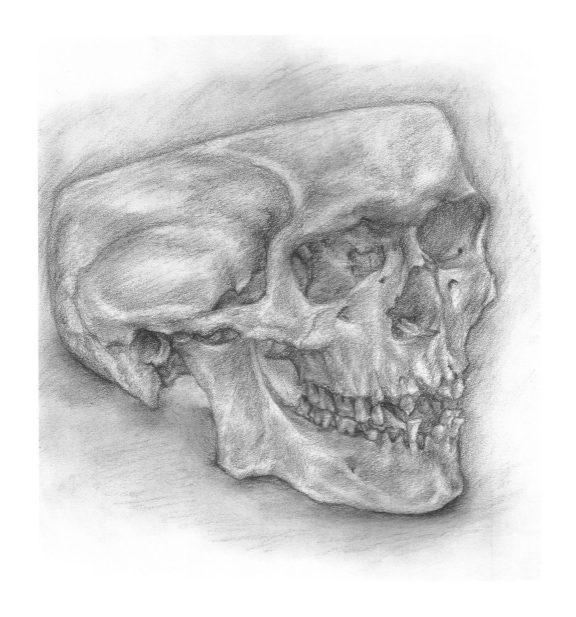

Zoe Marinides, Skull

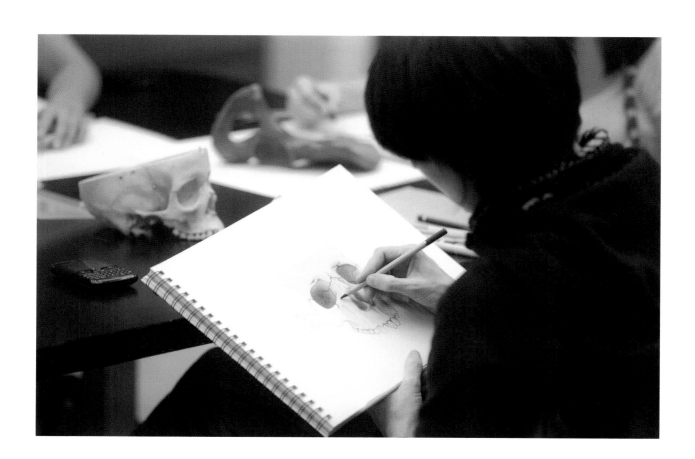

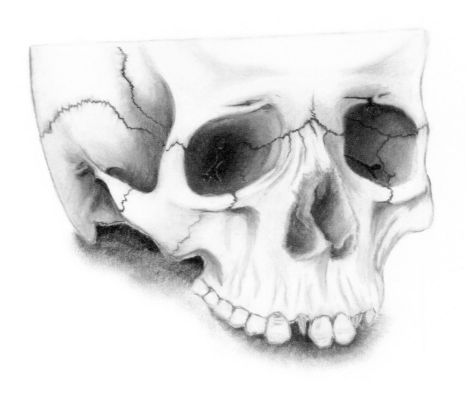

Sandrine Sanchez, Skull

"As a research scientist, I have great knowledge in biology and more specifically in cell biology. Art has always been a passion since childhood and getting the opportunity to combine Art & Anatomy was fantastic. I saw for the first time a fixed cadaver, fixed organs, I touched for the first time human bones and could observe with admiration how well built and structured they were."

– Sandrine Sanchez, PhD, Lab Supervisor, Neuroscience Institute

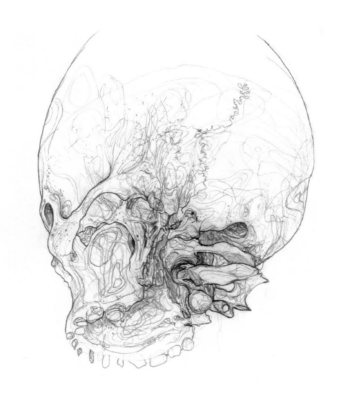

Yohei Rosen, Skull from below

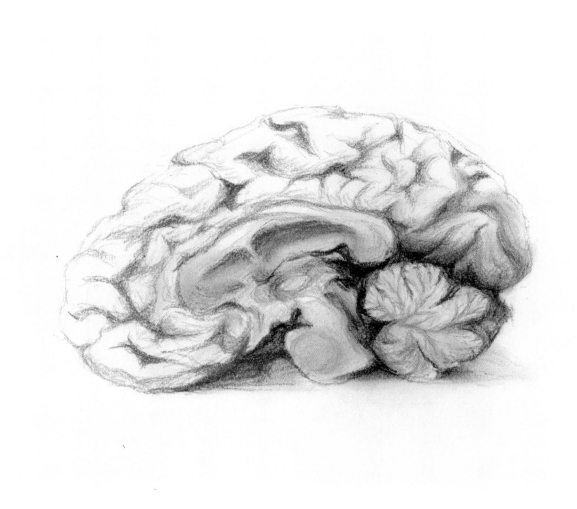

Ginny Bao, Brain

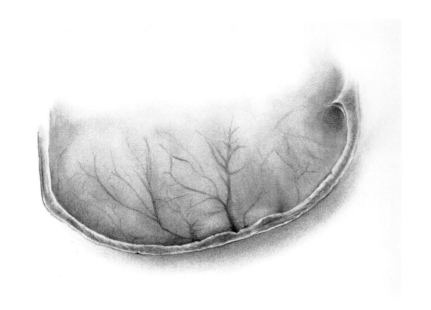

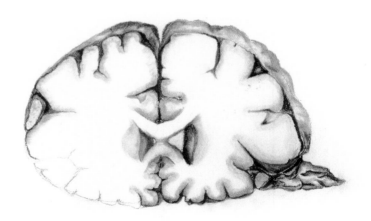

Silvia Curado, Inner skull with meningeal arteries (above) | Brain section (below)

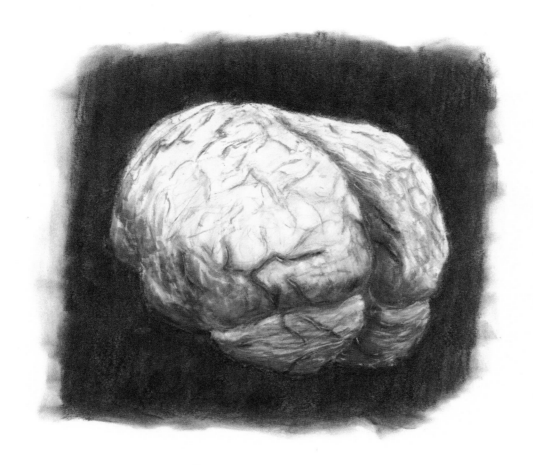

Adolfo Arias, Brain ("Interpretación del Cerebro")

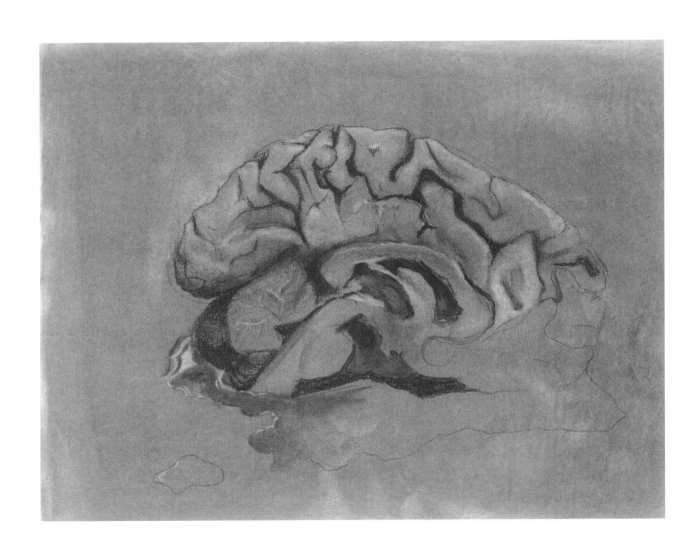

Kyra Edson, Brain

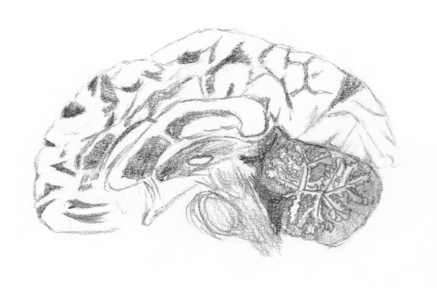

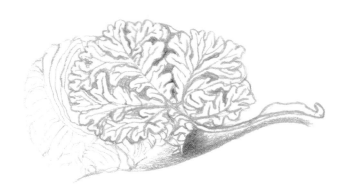

above: Marleigh Stern, Brain with cerebellum ("Brain Sketch") | below: Catherine Kulick, Cerebellum

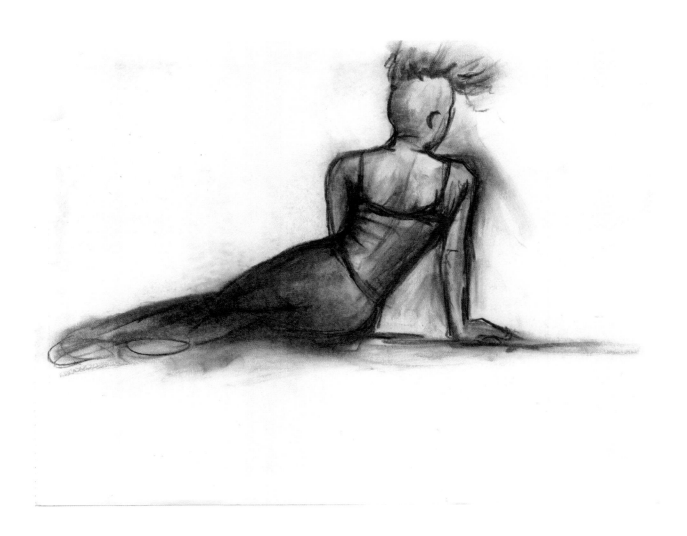

Hannah Bernstein, Model, stretched, leaning on arm

For one session we have life models come in to pose for us,
helping us to visually connect the body's inner space with its more familiar
exterior. We're thinking about movement. For some poses, we set up the
skeleton side by side with the model.

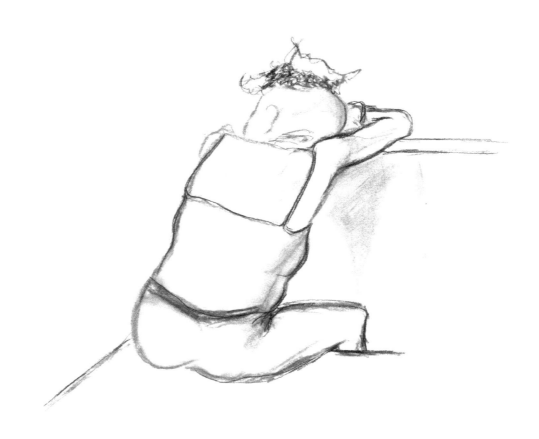

Amelie Pham, Life model ("Black Lines")

"This seminar was a nice way to let go of our role as students and let our brains be creative in a completely different way. As I relaxed, I let my mind wander and my hands draw out the stress, the emotions, the serenity, all the while enjoying a new connection with the anatomy models or cadavers that I attempted to draw."

– Amelie Pham, MD, class of 2016

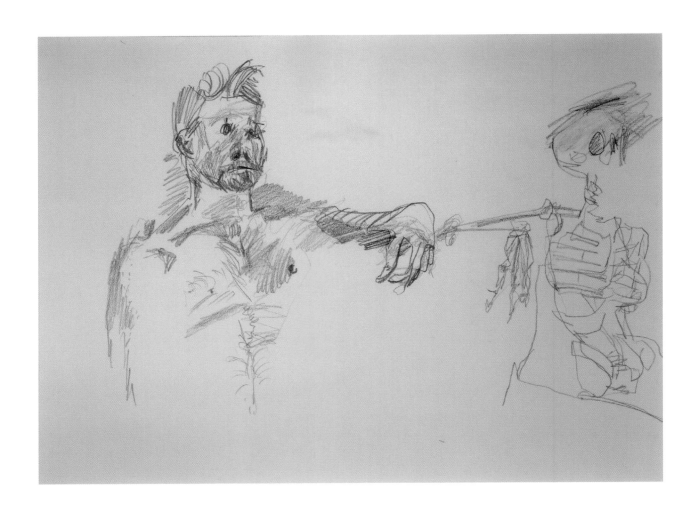

Michael Cammer, Model posing with skeleton

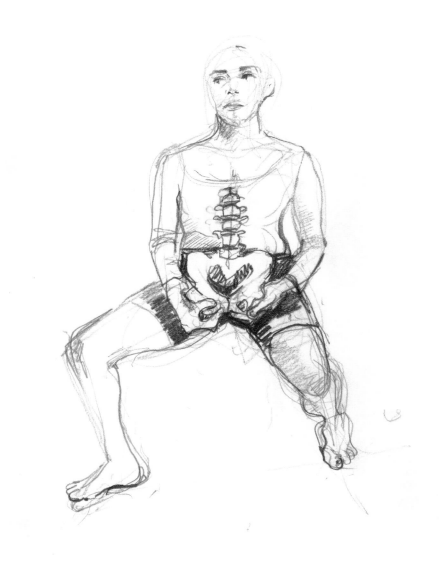

Cila Brosius, Model holding skeleton

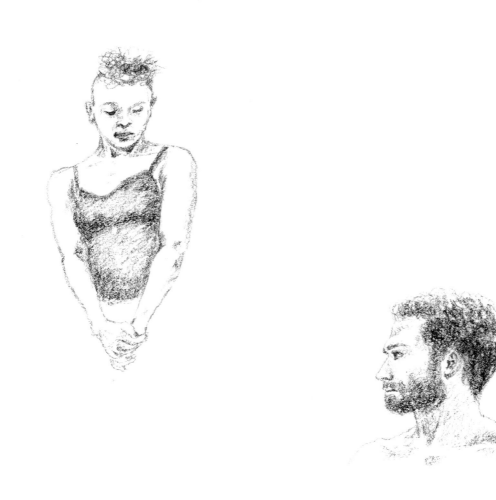

Shimwoo Lee, Model studies

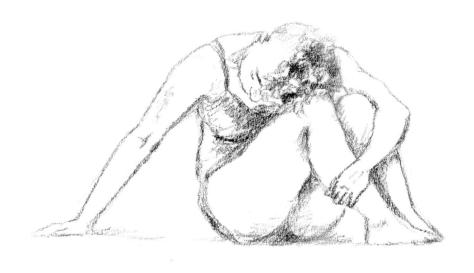

Shimwoo Lee, Life model study

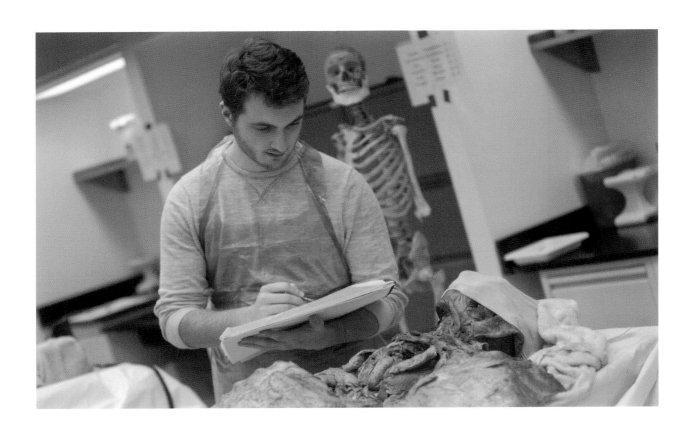

Drawing from the cadavers can be complicated and challenging
– artistically, logistically, and emotionally.

Dissection allows us to see the inner body in all its awesome complexity – art
lets us endow it with life. The details of bones and muscles tell a story of
movement and action, of life lived.

"Initially, the anatomy laboratory was a daunting place. Many of us had never seen a cadaver before, let alone dissected one. It was unsettling, to say the least. Through drawing, I was able to achieve a level of comfort in the lab that was previously elusive. It was as if changing the approach to them shifted the relationship we had with our cadavers."

– Aviva Regev, MD, class of 2012

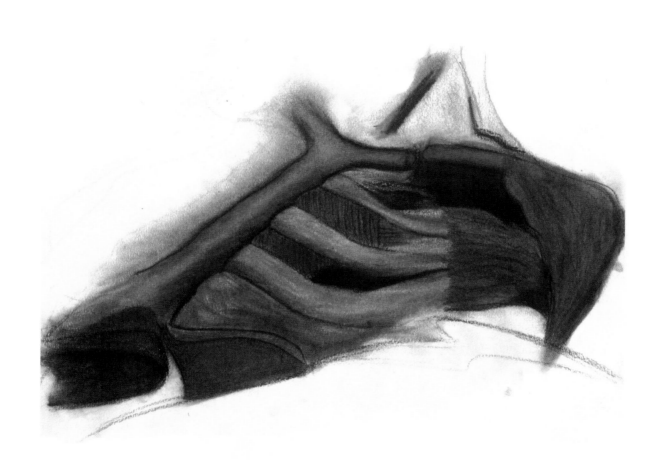

Aviva Regev, Cadaver ribcage ("Inside")

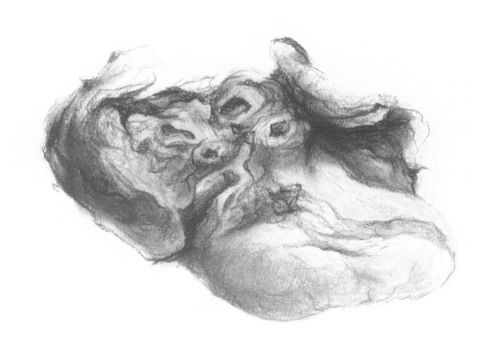

Ginny Bao, Chest cavity

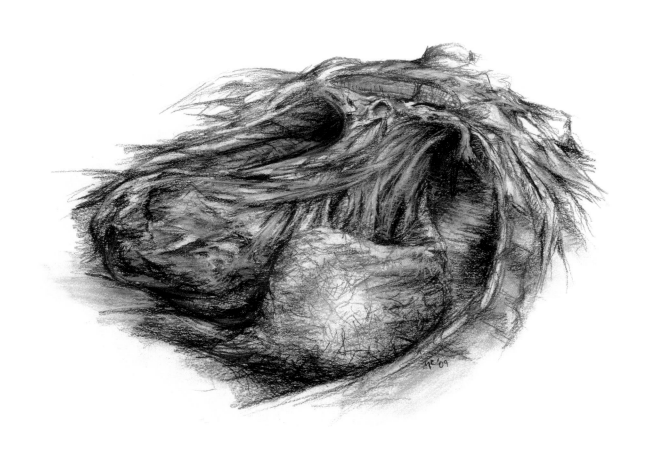

Michael Malone, Abdominal cavity ("Beds of Mussels and Whales")

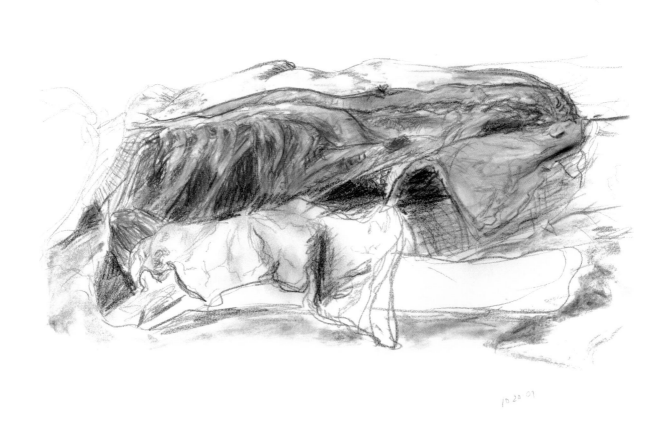

Karen M. Ong, Cadaver ("Under My Skin II")

"I am profoundly grateful for the opportunity to have had the chance to participate in the Art & Anatomy seminar in my first year of medical school. I had never before confronted death in any significant way and was apprehensive about human anatomy, which many consider a 'rite of passage' in becoming a physician. Participating in the drawing sessions in the anatomy lab gave me time to reflect and process my feelings about death, dying, and dissection prior to the start of the formal medical school anatomy course. For me, creating art is a meditative experience, and the Art & Anatomy course helped me take that mindfulness into the anatomy lab and find beauty in what otherwise would have been a highly distressing experience. After taking the course, I not only improved as an artist but also felt much more emotionally prepared to begin dissection."

– Karen M. Ong, class of 2018

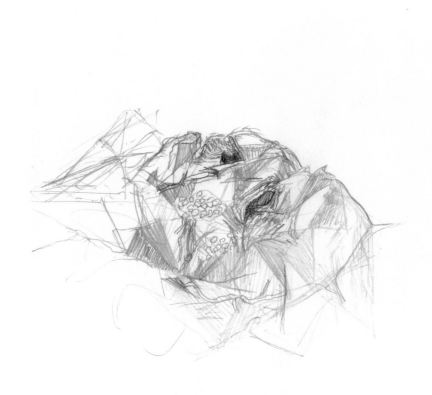

Yohei Rosen, Face of cadaver

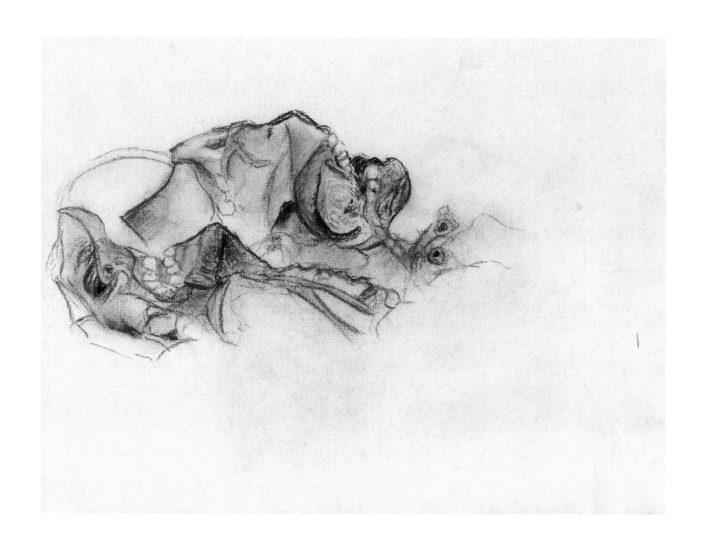

Karen M. Ong, Bisected head ("Inside My Head")

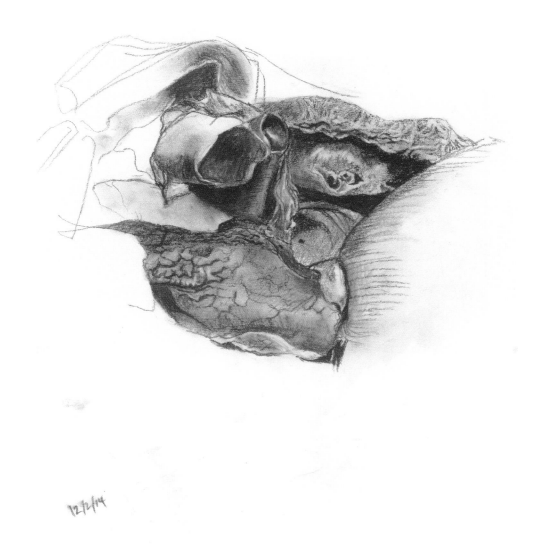

12/2/14

Kyra Edson, Thorax

"Art & Anatomy gives students time to appreciate their cadavers without the distraction of memorizing arteries, veins and nerves. Spending time in the lab without a testable task to accomplish offers time for reflection and appreciation of detail. When I sit in front of a cadaver with paper and pencil I am truly humbled by the complexity of the human body. A piece of tissue that might be torn away during dissection in search of a particular structure becomes equally important in the artist's eye as he or she draws that tissue in relation to the rest of the body."

– Kyra Edson, class of 2019

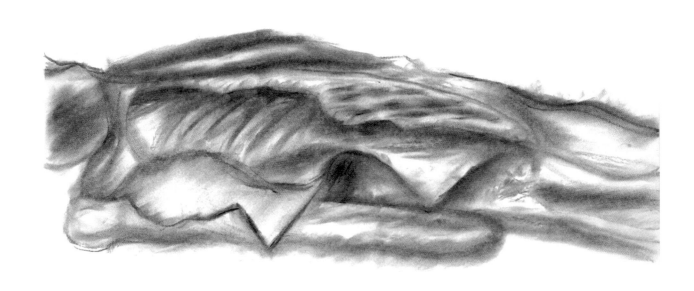

Nicholas Streicher, Cadaver on table ("Art & Anatomy")

"This course unifies what has been divided – and goes back to the origin of anatomy that began with drawings, in the era of early humanism, or return to the classics. As the practice of medicine becomes increasing mechanized, Art & Anatomy attempts to restore to medicine what is at risk to lose – an intellectual and creative experience that is at the core of medicine itself."

– Nicholas Streicher, MD, class of 2015

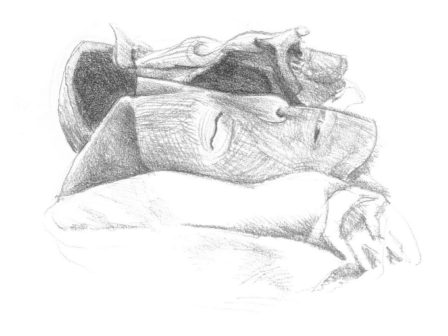

Jesse Kosskey, Head of cadaver

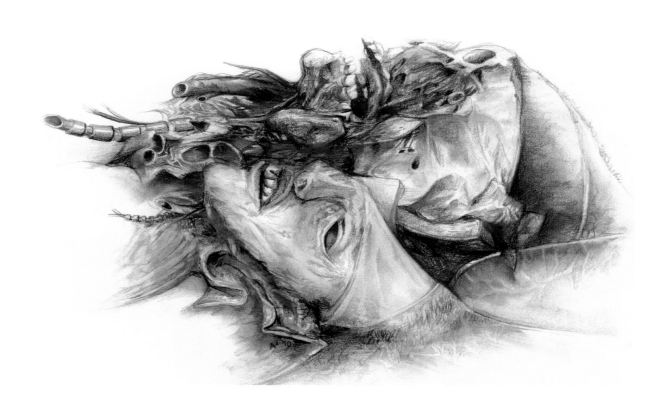

Michael Malone, Bisected head ("Abandon")

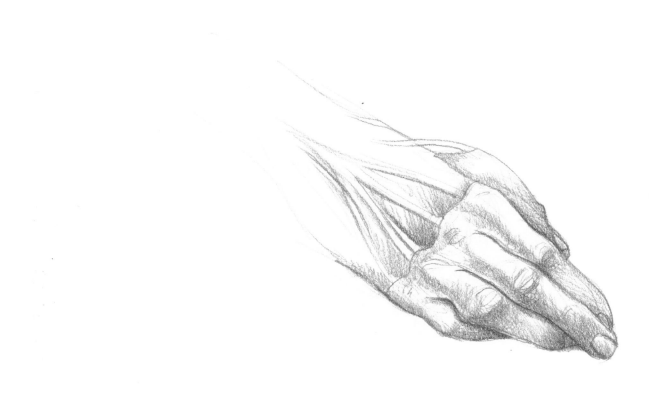

Jesse Kosskey, Hand with tendons

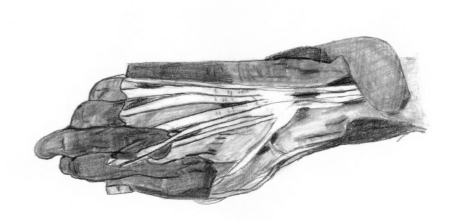

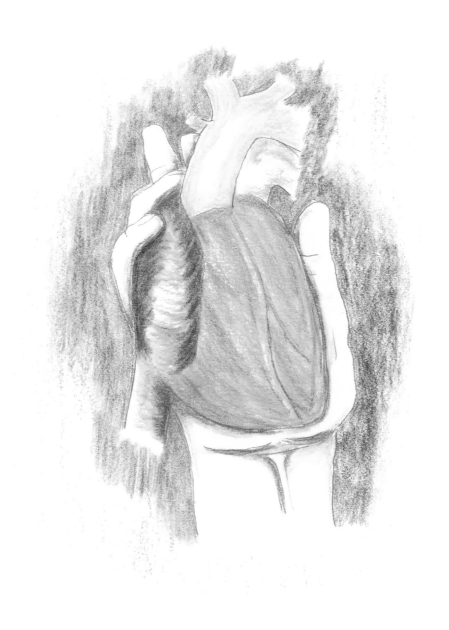

Abe DeAnda Jr., Heart in hand

For a closer look, we bring out organs that have been dissected from the cadavers, including the heart, kidney, liver, lung.

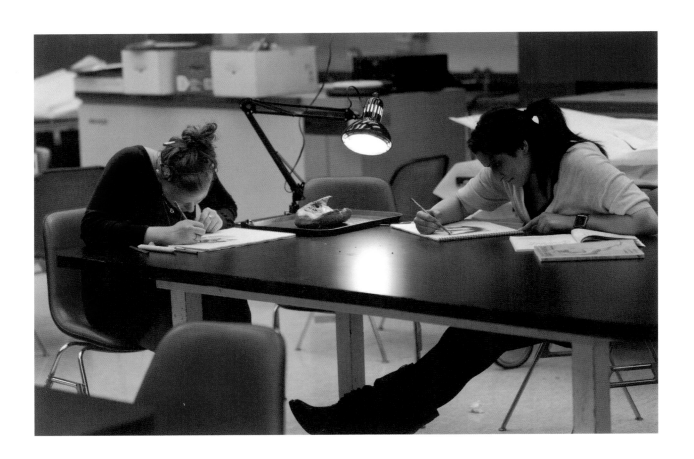

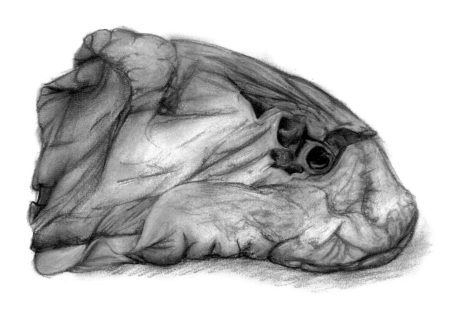

Hannah Bernstein, Lung

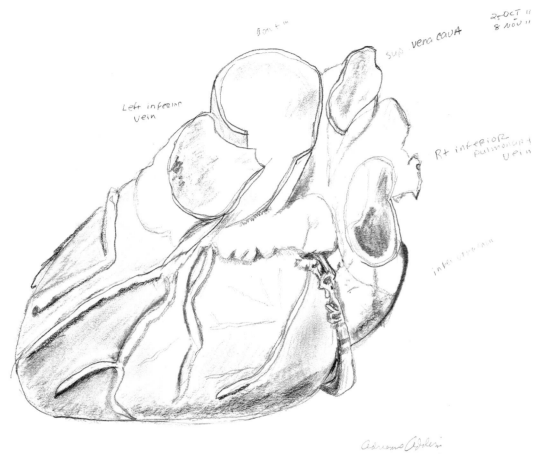

Adrienne Adessi, Heart

122

"The time just flew by in this class. You thought you saw every detail, but trying to draw makes you take a closer look, and more details would become evident."

– Adrienne Addessi, RN, MA, Faculty Group Practice Nurse,
Division of Hematology & Medical Oncology

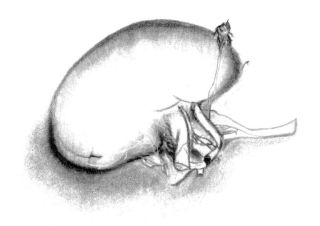

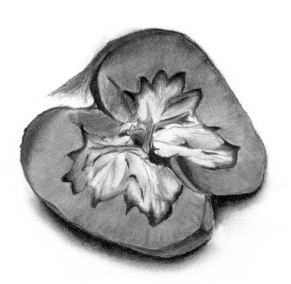

above: Kritika Nayar, Kidney ("The Ology of Kidneys") | below: Silvia Curado, PhD, Kidney, bisected

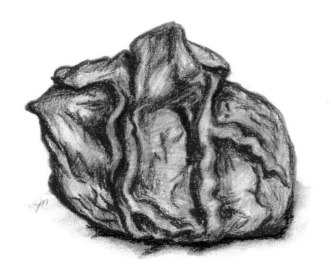

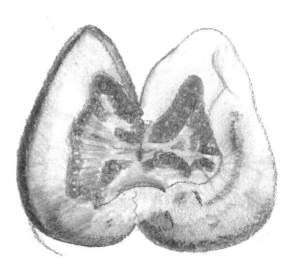

above: Jessica Meyer, Red heart ("Take to Heart") | below Yelena Sionova, Kidney, bisected

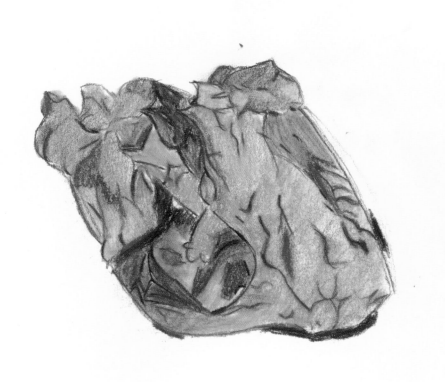

Akila Ramaraj, Inner heart

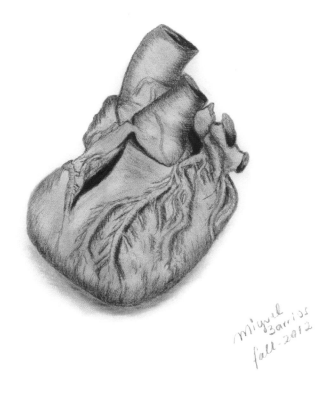

"That heart some days before was alive, pumping blood, then it was outside the body."

– Miguel Barrios-Barrios, MD, Research Coordinator,
Center for Healthful Behavior Changes

Miguel Barrios-Barrios, Heart ("A Drawing from the Heart")

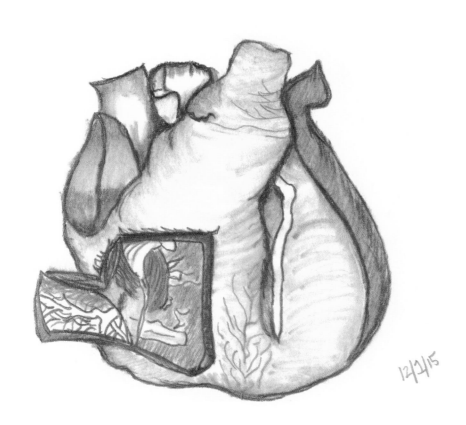

Pooja Patel, Heart ("Window into the Heart")

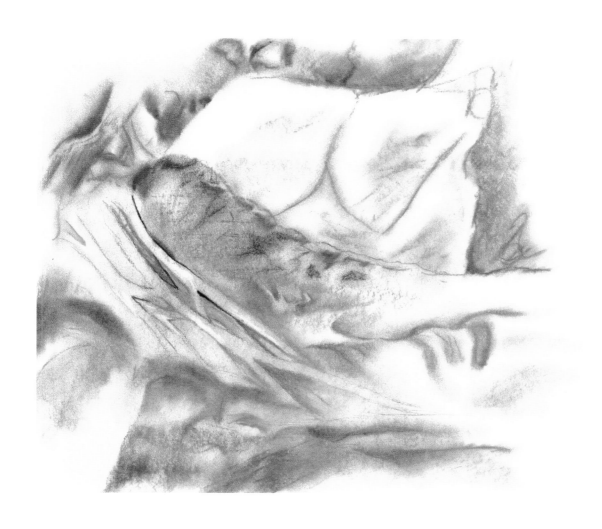

Jide Oluwadare, Brachial plexus ("Opened Chest")

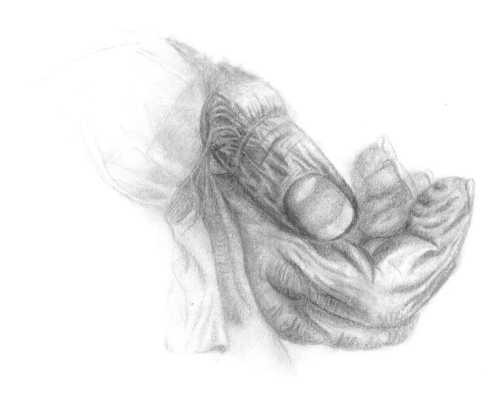

Shimwoo Lee, Cadaver hand with curled fingers

"How beautiful is a human body? Every detail of the human body – the contours of the muscle, the creases on the skin, and the curvatures of the bones – is a miraculous wonder of nature. For me, depicting the human body through art is a celebration of that beauty."

– Shimwoo Lee, MD, class of 2017

Art & Anatomy Curriculum

Laura Ferguson

One of the goals for this book is to inspire others to introduce anatomy drawing at their own medical schools and in pre-med programs around the country. So in this brief "how-to," I'll tell you more about how Art & Anatomy works on a session-by-session basis and how I function as facilitator/teacher. This is not meant as a script to be rigorously followed, but rather a springboard for your own ideas.

Art & Anatomy meets eight times over the course of one semester. Each session focuses on an issue or concept related to visualizing the inner body. Looking at related visual representations provides students with a chance to learn from other artists, and puts their own work in the historical context of the art of anatomy. Given the wide range of skill levels and drawing experience, students work at their own pace on aspects of artistic technique, with help from the facilitator. The majority of each 90-minute session is devoted to drawing.

Who could teach this class

My own background and skill set, as an artist who has been studying anatomy and making art about the inner body for over 25 years, is somewhat unique. But I know many others could facilitate such a class, bringing their own backgrounds and interests to the task. A love of drawing almost goes without saying. Beyond that, the main prerequisite is motivation – your own desire to learn, and the belief that learning itself is a creative process. Those who might teach Art & Anatomy include doctors or other medical professionals who love both drawing and anatomy; figurative artists who would be excited to have access to the Anatomy Lab; and perhaps medical illustrators, whose work already combines artistic skill with anatomical knowledge – though they'd need to take a looser approach to scientific accuracy.

Setting the stage: from Anatomy Lab to art studio

The first step is to set the stage for creativity – to establish the relaxed, creative atmosphere that will signal the intent to make art.

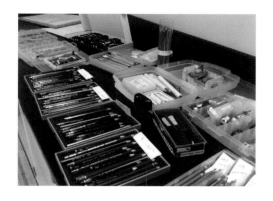

Art supplies   I'm a great believer in the idea that artists can do their best work when they find the right media, so I provide a wide variety of drawing materials: charcoal, graphite, color, and pastel pencils; Conté crayons; and felt-tip markers with brush and fine point. To encourage experimentation, I suggest artists keep a blank sheet in their pads for trying out materials and testing color combinations. Kneaded and rubber erasers, pencil sharpeners, and tortillons for blending and shading are also provided. Each student is given a drawing pad (Strathmore 400 series, medium surface, 11" x 14"), which will be theirs to keep. I have a selection of other papers on hand – larger sizes, smoother surfaces, and colors: brown kraft paper, tinted pastel and charcoal paper, and black paper for drawing in white from x-rays.

Book collection   We can learn so much by looking at what other artists have done and how they've handled various visual issues, especially when they've drawn the same bones or muscles we're working on. A small collection of books on anatomical art provides a historical context for the work we're doing. We have facsimile editions of Vesalius' and Albinus' anatomical atlases and Leonardo da Vinci's notebooks of anatomy drawings, a well as illustrated histories of anatomical art. There are no "how-to" books on anatomy drawing, but we have books on figure drawing technique that show the underlying anatomy as a framework for the figure.

Bulletin board   More visual references are provided by the prints I post on a large bulletin board in the Anatomy Lab. In the first years, when the class was just getting started, I posted images from the history of anatomical art, along with examples of my own work. Now the board is filled with drawings made in Art & Anatomy. It has become a resource for everyone who comes to the lab, and I often see med students and visitors spending time perusing the images.

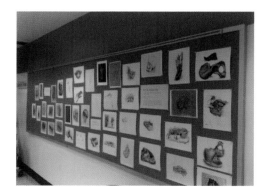

<u>Technique: getting it right vs. being expressive</u>

Medical students are used to having to get things right. They listen to lectures, study from textbooks, then are tested on how much they have memorized and understood. In medicine the answers are either right or wrong, and the stakes are high.

But art is not about right or wrong. In drawing it's good to experiment, to take risks – and the stakes here are very low. We want to make good drawings, of course, but making a great drawing doesn't necessarily mean a perfectly representational one. A perfect drawing may be boring: it can be hard to have a relationship with it. An imperfect (or unfinished) drawing might be the one viewers most enjoy looking at: they may have the same questions as the artist did, and enjoy sharing in the quest.

The class is open to all, and there's a wide range of drawing skill and experience; I talk briefly with each artist to evaluate their level. But I don't say much about drawing technique at the start. I prefer to let participants discover for themselves what the issues are: what questions they need to ask and what problems to solve. The single most important piece of advice I can give is to draw what you see – that is, don't over-think it or try to figure it out, just draw what you see in front of you. Our preconceptions can get in the way of seeing reality.

I tell the students that if they keep coming to class, their drawings will get better. Drawing is in large part a physical skill, and the development of eye-hand coordination can only be acquired by doing. I suggest some exercises, especially for beginners: for example, draw circles, then try using various shading techniques to turn them into spheres. It's a good way to loosen up the drawing hand, and helps us connect with the more intuitive side of the brain. And it's fun to be messy with art materials: working with charcoal or pastel, mistakes can be rubbed into the paper and become part of a textured background that adds to the sense of depth.

The central problem in drawing is making forms look three-dimensional on a two-dimensional surface, and shading is the key. There are no straight lines in the body, and I suggest that artists follow the curving natural forms in their shading. As their eyes get adjusted to seeing more details, they can see and follow the textured markings visible on the surfaces of the bones themselves.

As we work on each drawing, we alternate between getting it right (problem-solving, working out proportions) and being expressive (trying to convey the essence, the feeling, the poetry, of our subject). In Art & Anatomy, our focus is more on expressiveness than perfect accuracy: our intent is not to be medical illustrators but to convey a sense of the Anatomy Lab experience.

Session 1: Drawing bones - seeing individuality

At the first session, I invite each student to choose a bone from the boxes laid out on the tables, preferably one that intrigues and inspires them in some way. I make sure they know which bone they're drawing, and where it fits in on the skeleton. In this context the bones represent objects of visual fascination rather than facts to be memorized. I call their attention to the dynamics of bones: the spiraling forms that allow movement in many directions, and the surface textures that represent attachments of tendons and ligaments—marks of a life lived.

Introduction to the cadavers   First-year med students at NYUSOM start dissection in late November, so those who participate in Art & Anatomy in the Fall semester are getting their first introduction to the cadavers through drawing. The same is true for many of the staff members who take my class. So at our first session I take participants on a tour of the lab and show them the cadavers, which are laid out in two adjoining rooms. If there are med students in the group who have already begun dissection, I ask them to show the others their cadavers.

Session 2: Drawing our own hands
Drawing ourselves is a way of relating to anatomy more personally. At our second session, I ask students to try drawing a part of their own bodies, and the most accessible is the hand. It's easy to feel your own bones, and see some of your tendons and veins, just under the surface of the skin. Drawing yourself makes you aware of your own anatomy and of your hand as the means of drawing, the vehicle for self-expression.

   To make it easy for beginners, I suggest they put their hands down flat on the paper and trace around them to get the proportions, then fill in the bones. More experienced artists can draw their hands from more dynamic points of view.

Session 3: Focus on visual story-telling
At our third session, I show examples of artworks that tell visual stories, including contemporary artists making self-representations of disabled or unusual bodies (e.g. Frida Kahlo, Kiki Smith, Riva Lehrer, Marc Quinn, Hannah Wilke, Katherine Sherwood, Gary Schneider), and ask students to tell a story through drawing. It may be an imagined portrait of the person whose bone or cadaver they're drawing, or an aspect of their own body experience (a student dealing with a recent hand injury, for example), or an encounter with a patient (x-rays brought in from an internship in the Spine Lab). It

may be an exploration of the relationship between two bones that connect to each other at a joint, or a tableau of bones arranged to resemble a musical instrument. The titles some students give their drawings hint at stories or deeper meanings behind their work: "Under My Skin" for a cadaver in its bag, for example; "Of Breath and Bone" for a ribcage; or "May I Have This Dance?" for a pair of clasped skeleton hands.

Session 4: Drawing from the cadavers

Drawing from the cadavers presents artistic and logistical challenges in addition to the emotional ones discussed in my introduction. To make it easier to work in the cadaver rooms, easels or clipboards are available to support drawing pads, and baggies or small boxes to hold drawing materials. I encourage artists to form groups and draw together, to assist each other through the challenges. This is an extraordinary and unusual opportunity they've been given, one that many artists outside the medical world only wish they could have.

Unlike a bone, which is a discrete object that's easy to see in its entirety, each cadaver presents an overwhelming amount of fascinating detail, and an artist has to focus in on a small area, and figure out how to not include the rest. The complexity and beauty of the inner body will come into focus as they get more accustomed to looking. Finding the individual details of each body's unique anatomy will help to bring their drawings alive.

Session 5: Life drawing - focus on movement

To connect the inner anatomy with the human figures we see and know from the outside, we have life models come in to pose for us for one session. When possible, we pose the skeleton side by side with the model.

Drawing helps us to perceive anatomical structures more three-dimensionally and gain a clearer understanding of spatial relationships within the body. Connecting the inner body to its exterior reminds us to see the whole person: a living, moving human body. We look at the work of artists like Auguste Rodin and Edgar Degas who often drew the figure, to learn from their techniques for evoking the dynamics of movement.

These life drawing sessions are a complete change of pace. We start with quick poses (one minute, five minutes), to get warmed up and to get familiar with the figure in general and these models in particular. Even our longer poses (10-15 minutes) are brief compared to our experience of drawing the bones or cadavers. This is a very different kind of session … all about movement.

Session 6: Drawing from anatomical specimens - heart, lung, liver, or kidney

To draw from anatomical specimens in more detail, we bring organs that have been dissected out from the cadavers into the study room to draw. Students help to remove and detach organs from the cadavers, and in the process gain a sense of their spatial relationship to the whole. Materials such as blocks of styrofoam are available to help position specimens at best angles, and pins to prop them open so inner structures are visible. Our focus here is on drawing the details. Hearts are the most popular subject, lungs and livers are also available, and the insides of bisected kidneys turn out to be surprisingly beautiful.

Session 7: Drawing the brain

Medical students at NYUSOM don't dissect the brain; they learn about and observe brain specimens in the neuroanatomy lab. For one session I arrange for my Art & Anatomy students to draw from brain specimens in the neuroanatomy lab: whole brains, hemispheres, and coronal sections. It's probably our most awe-inspiring session, and many wonderful drawings are made.

Brain tissue, made up almost entirely of nerves, is different from other types of body tissue. We focus on the details of brain structure. In the whole brains and hemispheres, we notice that the pattern of folds is unique to each individual. In the coronal sections, we notice and draw the patterns created by the differences in coloration between gray matter and white matter.

Session 8: Finishing drawings

Our final session is a time to finish up drawings in progress or a last chance to draw something new. We get to take a look at each other's work. I look through students' pads and help them choose which drawings to have scanned, which makes them available for future projects like exhibitions, posting on the bulletin board, or submitting to the student magazine, *Agora*.

As they leave, I urge these artists to keep drawing – and at that moment, feeling inspired, they all vow that they will. I hope it's true, and look forward to finding out in future years about the impact Art & Anatomy has had on their lives as medical professionals.

About the Contributors

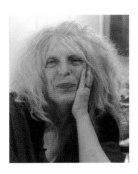

Laura Ferguson is Artist in Residence in the Master Scholars Program in Humanistic Medicine at NYU School of Medicine, where she created the Art & Anatomy seminar. She is Art Editor of the *Literature, Arts and Medicine Database*. Laura became interested in anatomy because of her own curvature of the spine, and has made her body and its anatomy the subject of her art. Her drawings and prints have been featured in seminal exhibitions on art and medicine, including "Seeing Ourselves" at MuseCPMI in New York, "Humans Being" at the Chicago Cultural Center, and "Beyond the X-ray" at the Museum of Science in Boston. Her "Visible Skeleton" series was featured at the National Museum of Health and Medicine in Washington DC, and her work is in the collections of the National Library of Medicine and the American Academy of Orthopaedic Surgeons. To see more: www.lauraferguson.net

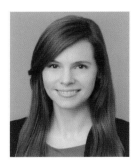

Katie Grogan, DMH, MA is Associate Director of the Master Scholars Program in Humanistic Medicine and Adjunct Instructor of Medical Humanities at NYU School of Medicine. She holds a Bachelor's Degree in English and American Literature and a Master's Degree in Humanities and Social Thought, both from NYU, as well as a Doctorate in Medical Humanities from Drew University. She develops curricular and co-curricular programming at the intersections of medicine with the arts, humanities, and social sciences to enhance the experiences of students and the wider community of NYU School of Medicine.

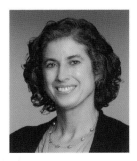

Danielle Ofri, MD, PhD is an internist at Bellevue Hospital and Associate Professor of Medicine at NYU School of Medicine, as well as Editor-in-Chief of the Bellevue Literary Review. She writes regularly for the *New York Times, Slate Magazine*, and other publications about medicine and the doctor-patient relationship. Ofri is the author of five books about life in medicine. Her most recent book is *What Patients Say; What Doctors Hear*.

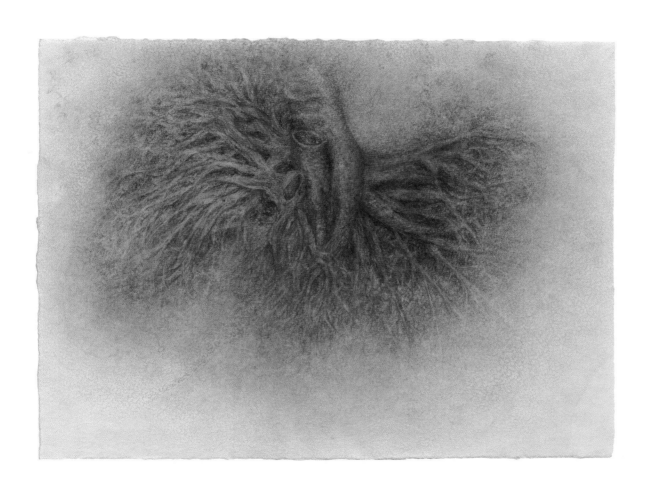

Laura Ferguson, "Lung, opened"

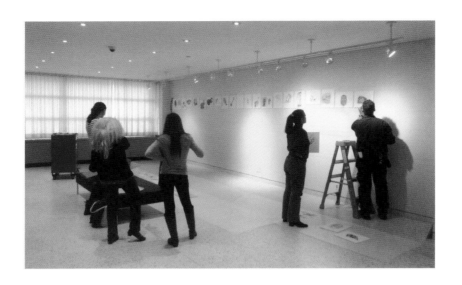

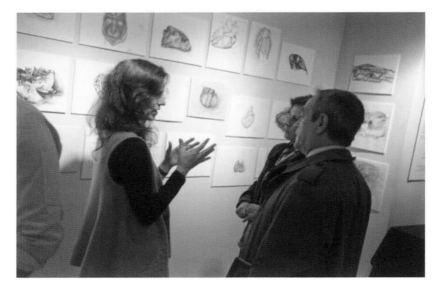

"Art & Anatomy: Drawings" exhibit in NYU Langone's art gallery, January 2014
above: installing the art | below: the opening reception

Acknowledgments

Front cover artwork: Hannah Bernstein, "Open Heart"

Photographs of the class and the gallery exhibition:
Andrew Neary (pages 6, 38, 45, 48, 53, 66, 83, 100, and back cover),
Alan Barnett (pp. 12, 22, 80, 120), Olivia Smith (p. 24), and Tiffany Cook (p. 133),
for NYULMC; Silvia Curado (p. 140, top)
Contributor photos (p. 138): top, Emon Hassan (still from video "How to Draw a Human
Heart"); center, Jeff Weiner; bottom, NYU staff

Book design: Laura Ferguson

Thanks to the Office of Student Affairs and the Master Scholars Program in Humanistic
Medicine, especially:
Linda Tewksbury, MD, Associate Dean for Student Affairs
David Oshinsky, PhD and Michael Tanner, MD, Faculty Co-Directors

Thanks to Master Scholars Program graduate assistants Tamara Prevatt and Song Eun We,
and Project Associate Sasha Kruger, for their help with this book.

Thanks to George Lew and Terrance Fell for their help every week in the Anatomy Lab, and
to the faculty and staff of the Departments of Cell Biology and Pathology for their knowledge
and expertise.

Thanks to all the artists who have come to draw, and allowed us to show their work.
Thanks especially to those who have donated their bodies to the Anatomy Lab, and allowed
us to learn.

Artists who were medical students when they participated in Art & Anatomy

Each drawing has a simple, anatomically descriptive title; some artists also added their own titles.

Artists who were faculty or staff of NYU School of Medicine/ NYU Langone Medical Center

Abe DeAnda Jr., MD, Associate Professor, Cardiothoracic Surgery — Heart in hand 118
Adolfo Arias, Spanish Medical Interpreter, Language Access Services Department
— Brain ("Interpretación del Cerebro") 89
Adrienne Addessi, RN, MA, FGP Nurse, Division of Hematology & Medical Oncology — Heart 122
Alejandra Yancey, Student — Femur studies 44
Ariana Ilene Rabinowitsch, Associate Research Technician, Department of Psychiatry — Humerus ("Long Bone") 69
Arlene Paul, Medical Coder — Pelvis 50
Cila Brosius, Graduate Student, Visual Arts Administration, NYU Steinhardt — Model holding skeleton 97
David Fooksman, Assistant Professor of Pathology, Albert Einstein College of Medicine — Pelvis with hip joints 40
Harold Horowitz, MD, Professor of Medicine, Infectious Diseases and Immunology, Bellevue Hospital Center
— Box of bones 21
— Hanging skeleton 26
Jesse Koskey, MD, Resident, NYU Department of Psychiatry — Head of cadaver 114
— Hand with tendons 116
Kella L. Vangsness, Associate Researcher, NYU Hospital for Joint Diseases — Hand with hand skeleton 74
Kritika Nayar, Clinical Psychology Graduate Student, Northwestern Feinberg School of Medicine
— Kidney ("The Ology of Kidneys") 124
Kyle Anthony Durrant, Project Associate, Office of Medical Education — Skeleton hand ("The Hand") 70
Kyra Doumlele, Research Coordinator — Hand with skeleton 75
Linnea Russell, Research Assistant — Pelvis with sketches 41
Michael Cammer, Research Associate, Microscopy, OCS — Pelvis study 51
— Model posing with skeleton 96
Miguel Barrios-Barrios, MD, Research Coordinator, Center for Healthful Behavior Changes
— Heart ("A Drawing from the Heart") 127
Sandrine Sanchez, PhD, Lab Supervisor, Neuroscience Department — Skull 84
Silvia Curado, PhD, Faculty — Ribs with light shining through 37
— Inner skull with meningeal arteries | Brain section 88
— Kidney, bisected 124
Valeria Mezzano, Research Scientist, Leon Charney Division of Cardiology — Foot 55
Wendy Agudo, Communications and Strategies Specialist — Humerus ("Mechanics of the Body") 72
Yelena Sionova, Director of Research Administration, Department of Medicine — Kidney, bisected 125